HEALTHY EATING COOKBOOK

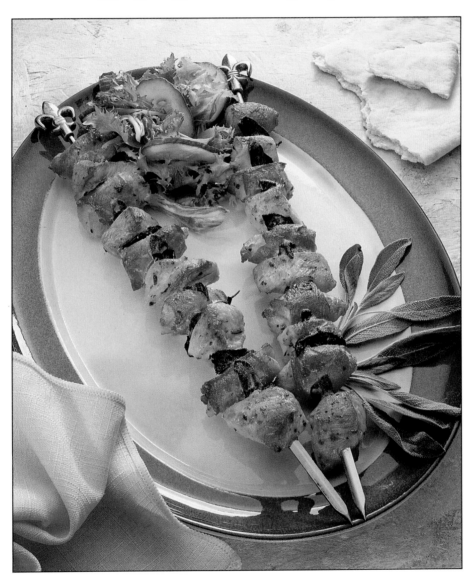

Designed by Sally Strugnell and Claire Leighton
Illustrations by Christine Berrington
Food photography by Peter Barry
Edited by Ros Cocks, Jillian Stewart and
Kate Cranshaw

CLB 3281
All rights reserved.
This 1993 edition published by Magna Books,
Magna Road, Wigston, Leicester LE18 4ZH.
© 1993 Colour Library Books Ltd., Godalming,
Surrey, England.
Printed and bound in Singapore.
ISBN 1 85422 506 5

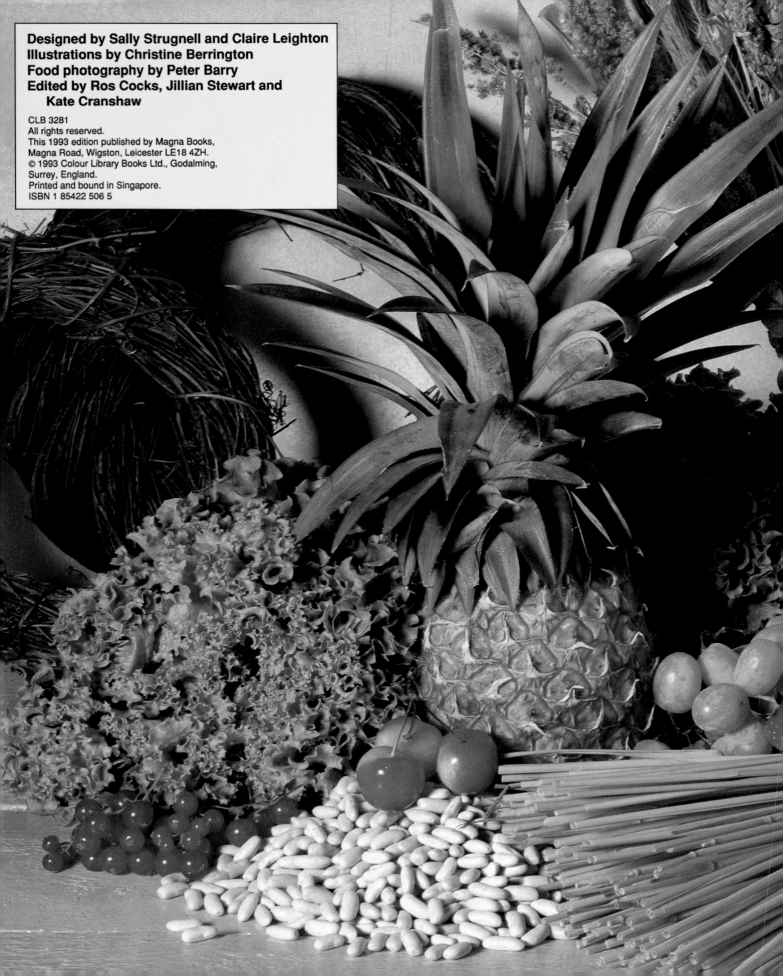

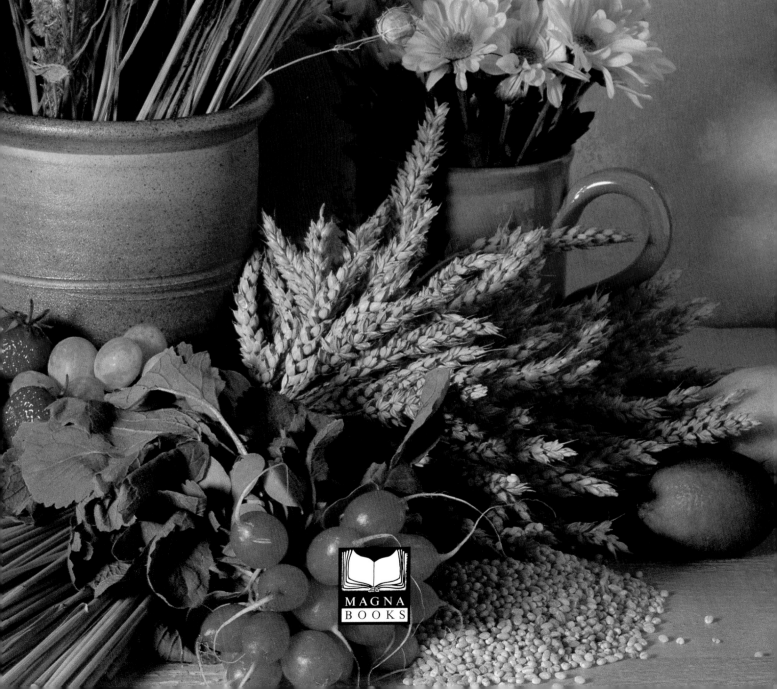

HEALTHY EATING
COOKBOOK

MAGNA BOOKS

INTRODUCTION

Health consciousness has increased dramatically over the past 50 years to such an extent that today you are considered almost irresponsible if you are overweight, a smoker, or just generally unfit. Food is no longer seen as simply something to satisfy hunger, but as a vital element in a healthy lifestyle. And indeed, it has become generally accepted that two of the main factors affecting health are diet and exercise.

Medical opinions – mainstream and fringe – regarding diet have varied over the last few decades, but these viewpoints are currently in broad agreement on certain basic guidelines. These generally advise you to eat plenty of fresh fruit and vegetables; ensure a good supply of fibre such as that found in wholemeal bread; eat a variety of different protein sources such as fish, chicken and pulses, as well as meat and dairy produce; and finally, limit your daily intake of fats, salt and sugar.

The argument against a high cholesterol intake continues, and it would be a brave person who could claim certainty regarding the benefits and disadvantages of unsaturated and saturated fats. At the present time semi-skimmed and skimmed milks, sunflower margarine and oil, and olive oil have the thumbs up, and it is thought that those at risk from heart disease should avoid full-cream milk, butter, cream and high-fat cheeses. If you are a regular meat eater it is now recognized that white meats, fish and the leaner cuts of red meat are ideal for avoiding an excessive intake of fats. Fatty meats, such as pork and lamb, are best eaten in moderation, or at least eaten complemented by plenty of fresh salads and vegetables. Chicken, turkey, veal, and white fish are all safe bets for a low-fat, high-protein diet.

When weighing up the pros and cons of different foods you should give just as much consideration to the method of cooking as to the ingredients. Always bear in mind that fresh, uncooked fruit and vegetables contain far more vitamins and minerals than their cooked counterparts. In order to maintain the vitamin content of these foods prepare them at the last minute and cook them for only a short time. Overcooking, or leaving fruit and vegetables to soak in water, should be avoided as this leaches them of vitamins. When cooking foods, try to grill rather than fry and if you must fry, add as little fat as possible. Try to avoid deep-fried foods, and if you are deep frying use sunflower oil and not lard. Barbecuing, like grilling, is an excellent method for cooking meat as this enables any excess fat to run off. Stir-frying of vegetables is also very good as only a little oil is required and the cooking is short, therefore retaining more of the nutrients.

Healthy cooking tastes good and is good for you. The recipes in this book are bright, cheerful and colourful. Soups, dips, salads, low-fat meat, fish and vegetable dishes are included, in addition to fruity puddings. Fun and simple to make, the recipes are well laid out and easy to follow, and with recipe ideas from many countries you will never stuck for ideas.

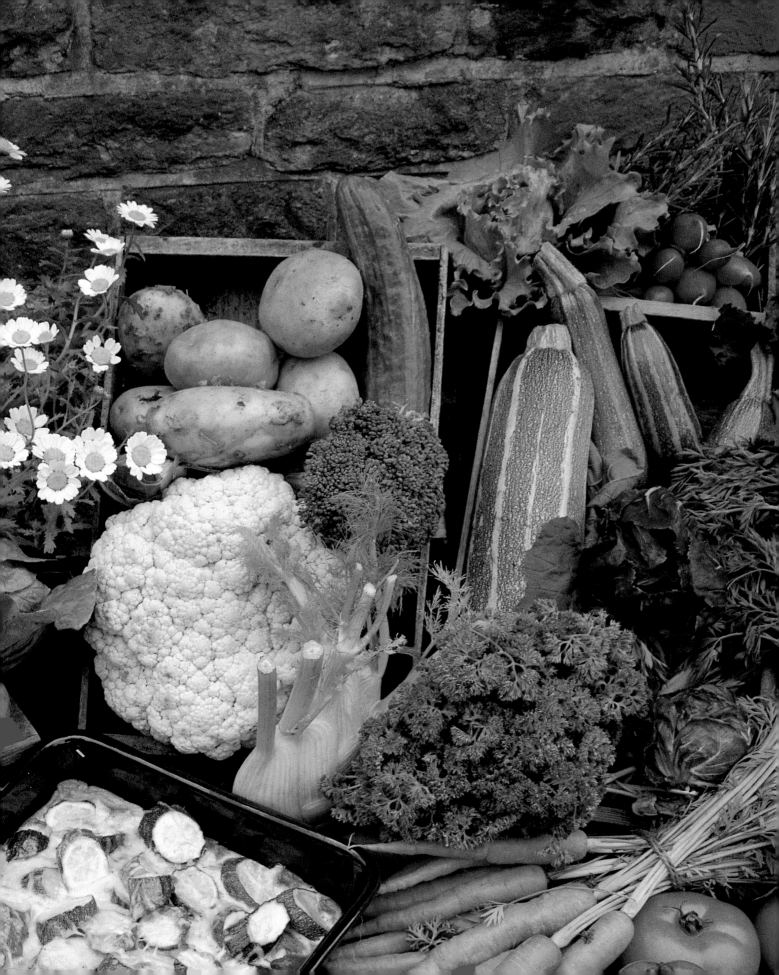

Minestrone Soup

Preparation Time: about 20 minutes, plus overnight soaking for the beans **Cooking Time:** 1½ hours **Serves:** 6

There are numerous different recipes for minestrone. This one is high in fibre and it has hardly any saturated fats at all.

Ingredients

120g/4oz dried white cannellini beans
1150ml/2 pints vegetable stock
2 tbsps olive oil
1 large onion, finely chopped
1 clove garlic, crushed
1 stick celery, thinly sliced
2 carrots, diced
120g/4oz spring greens, finely shredded
60g/2oz cut green beans
1 large courgette, diced
120g/4oz tomatoes, peeled, seeded and diced
1 bay leaf
60g/2oz wholemeal pasta
Salt and pepper
1 tbsp fresh chopped basil
1 tbsp fresh chopped parsley

Put the beans into a large bowl and cover with the vegetable stock. Leave to soak overnight. During this time the beans will double in volume.

Heat the oil in a large saucepan and gently fry the onion and garlic until they have softened, but not browned. Stir in the celery, carrots, spring greens, green beans and courgettes. Fry gently, stirring until they have just begun to soften. Add the beans with the stock to the pan of vegetables, along with the tomatoes, bay leaf, pasta and seasoning. Bring to the boil, then cover and simmer for about 1 hour, or until the beans are very tender. Stir occasionally during this time to prevent the ingredients from sticking. Stir in the basil and parsley, heat through for 5 minutes and serve immediately.

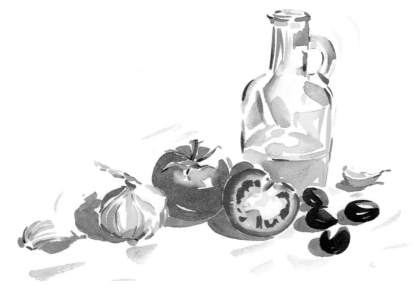

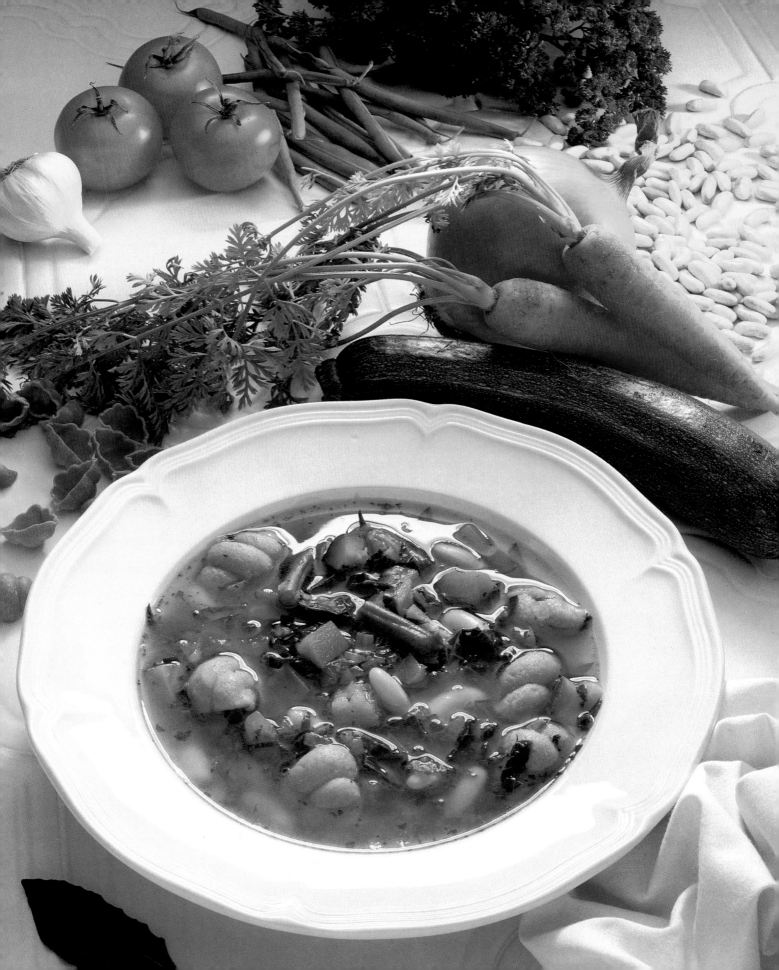

Taramasalata

Preparation Time: 15-25 minutes, plus 30 minutes chilling **Serves:** 4

This well known, classic Greek dip is a delicious starter eaten with warm pitta bread.

Ingredients
90g/3oz smoked cod roe
6 slices white bread, crusts removed
1 lemon
1 small onion, finely chopped

6 tbsps olive oil
Black olives and chopped fresh
   parsley, for garnish

Cut the cod roe in half and scrape out the centre into the bowl. Discard the skin. Put the bread into a bowl along with 140ml/¼ pint warm water. Allow the bread to soak for about 10 minutes, then drain off the water and squeeze the bread until it is almost dry. Add the bread to the bowl containing the cod roe. Squeeze the lemon and add the juice to the bread and roe, stirring it well. Liquidize the cod roe mixture with the onion until the ingredients form a smooth paste.

   Return the blended cod roe mixture to a bowl and gradually beat in the oil, a little at a time, as if making mayonnaise. Beat the mixture very thoroughly between additions with a whisk or wooden spoon. Refrigerate the taramasalata for at least ½ hour to chill thoroughly. Transfer the mixture to a serving bowl and garnish with the black olives and chopped parsley.

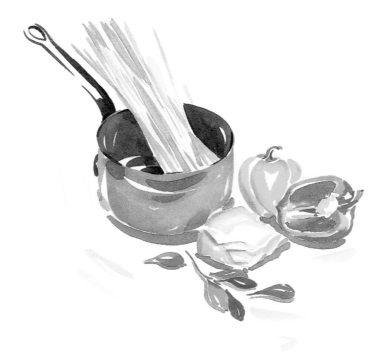

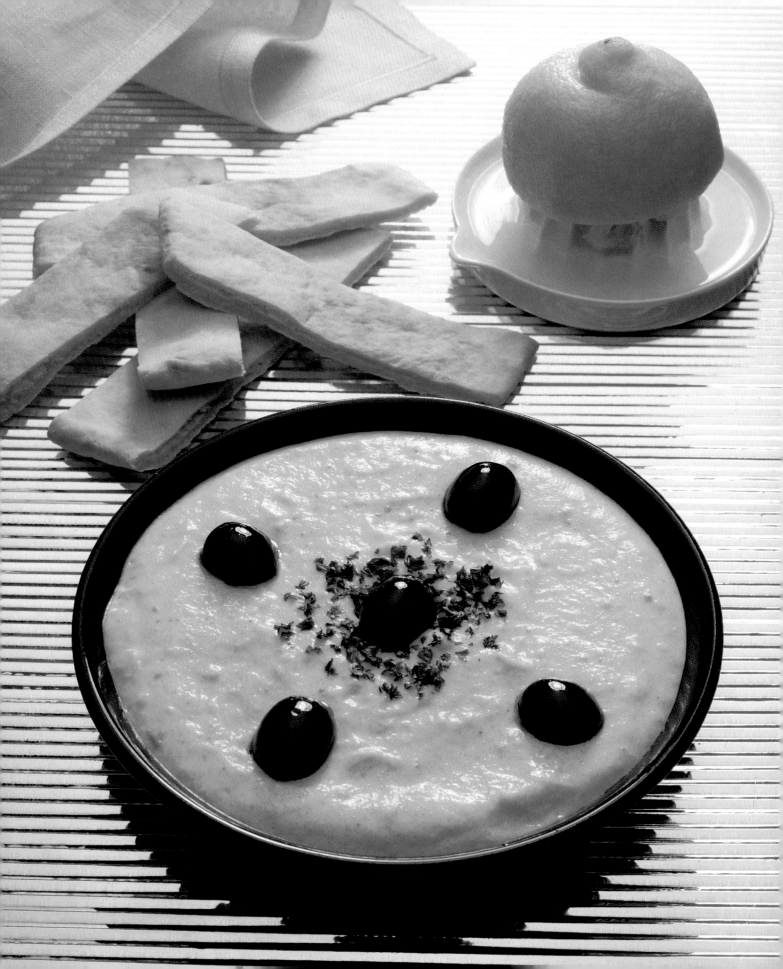

Watercress Soup

Preparation Time: 15 minutes **Cooking Time:** 45 minutes **Serves:** 4

Watercress is packed with vitamins and makes delicious soup.

Ingredients
60g/2oz butter
1 leek, thinly sliced
225g/8oz potatoes, thinly sliced
570ml/1 pint chicken stock
Pinch grated nutmeg
Salt and pepper

4 good bunches of watercress,
  washed and trimmed
3 tbsps cream
Few extra sprigs of watercress for
  garnish

Melt the butter in a large saucepan and gently cook the leek until it is just soft, stirring frequently to prevent it from browning. Add the potatoes, stock, nutmeg and seasoning to the saucepan. Bring to the boil, then cover and simmer for 15 minutes. Add the watercress and simmer for a further 10 minutes.

Cool the soup slightly, then liquidize the vegetables until very finely chopped. Rinse the saucepan and stand a fine meshed sieve over the cleaned pan.

Push the soup through the sieve using the back of a wooden spoon, working the watercress and vegetables through the mesh until only the tough stalks remain and the soup in the pan is a fine purée. Adjust the seasoning and stir the cream into the soup. Reheat gently, taking care not to boil it. Serve garnished with the reserved watercress sprigs and a little cream if desired.

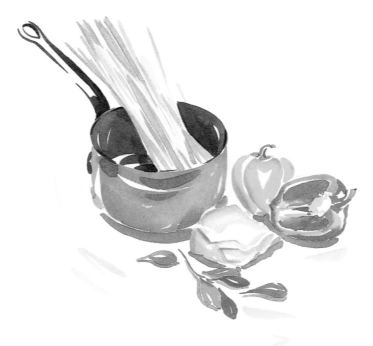

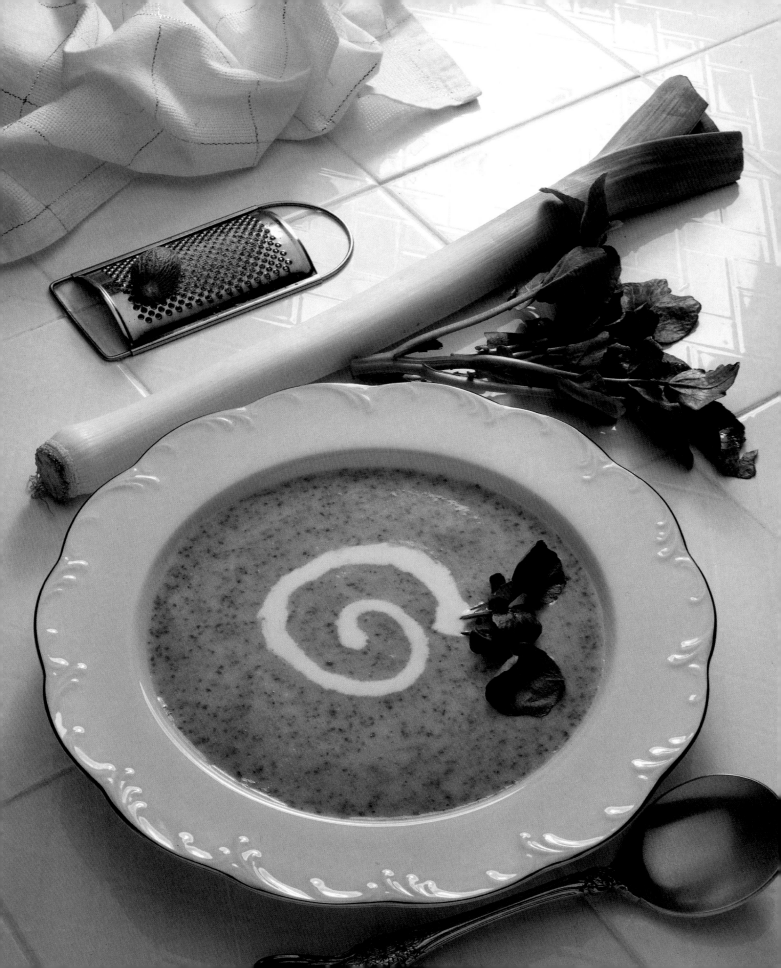

Terrine of Spinach and Chicken

Preparation Time: 25 minutes **Cooking Time:** 1 hour **Serves:** 6-8

This superb terrine is ideal when you want to impress your guests with a delicious appetizer.

Ingredients
225g/8oz chicken breasts, boned and skinned
2 egg whites
120g/4oz fresh white breadcrumbs
450g/1lb fresh spinach, washed
1 tbsp each of fresh finely chopped chervil, chives and tarragon

Freshly ground black pepper
280ml/½ pint double cream
60g/2oz finely chopped walnuts
Pinch of nutmeg

Cut the chicken into small pieces. Put the cut chicken, 1 egg white and half of the breadcrumbs into a food processor. Liquidize until well mixed. Remove from processor and rinse the bowl. Season the chicken mixture with a little pepper and add half of the cream. Mix well to blend thoroughly.

Put the spinach into a large saucepan and cover with a tight-fitting lid. Cook the spinach for 3 minutes, or until it has just wilted. Put the spinach into the food processor along with the herbs, the remaining egg white and bread-crumbs. Liquidize until smooth. Add the remaining cream to the spinach along with the walnuts and the nutmeg. Beat this mixture well to blend thoroughly.

Line a 450g/1lb loaf tin with greaseproof paper. Lightly oil this with a little vegetable oil. Pour the chicken mixture into the base of the tin and spread evenly. Carefully pour the spinach mixture over the chicken mixture, and smooth the top with a palette knife. Cover the tin with lightly oiled aluminium foil and seal this tightly around the edges. Stand the tin in a roasting dish and pour enough warm water into the dish to come halfway up the sides of the tin. Cook the terrine in a preheated oven 160°C/325°F/Gas Mark 3 for 1 hour, or until it is firm. Put the terrine into the refrigerator and chill for at least 12 hours.

Carefully lift the terrine out of the tin and peel off the paper. To serve, cut the terrine into thin slices with a sharp knife.

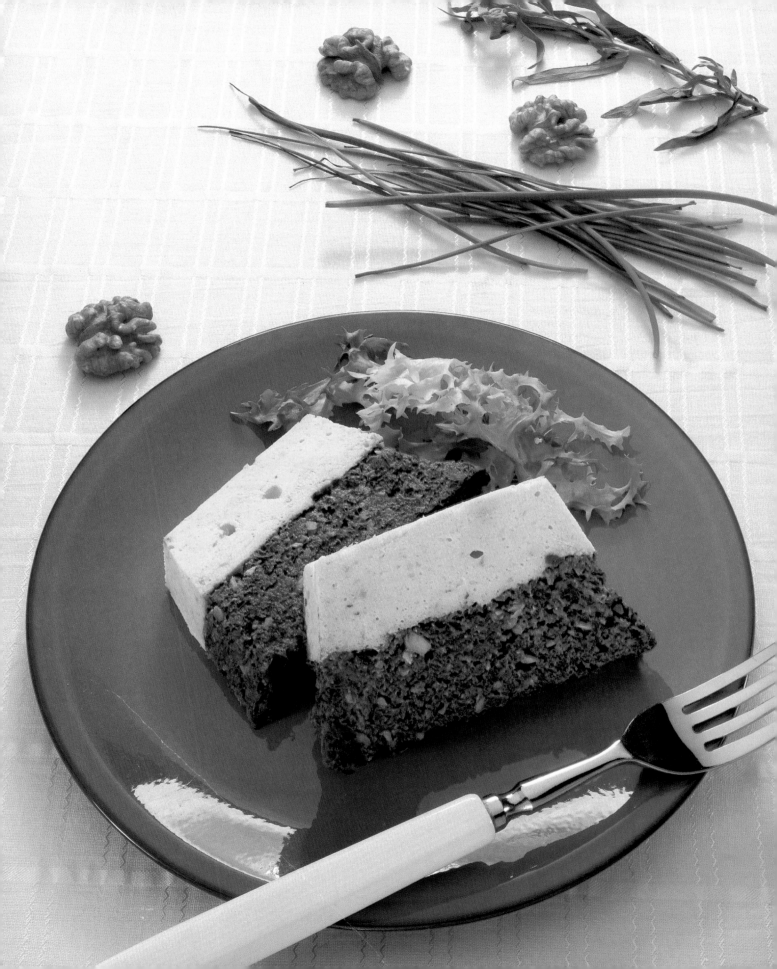

Courgette Soup with Lemon

Preparation Time: 20 minutes **Cooking Time:** 25 minutes **Serves:** 4-6

The fresh taste of lemon and courgettes makes a delicious soup which can be served either hot or cold.

Ingredients

1 medium-sized onion, thinly sliced
2 tbsps olive oil
450g/1lb courgettes, sliced
Finely grated rind and juice of 1 large
    lemon

430ml/¾ pint chicken stock
Freshly ground black pepper
2 egg yolks
200ml/⅓ pint natural yogurt

In a large pan, fry the onion gently in the olive oil for 3 minutes until it is just transparent.
    Add the courgettes and fry for a further 2-3 minutes. Stir in all remaining ingredients except the egg yolks and yogurt, cover and simmer for 20 minutes.
    Liquidize the soup until smooth. Mix the egg yolks into the yogurt and stir into the blended soup. Reheat the soup gently, stirring all the time until it thickens. Serve hot at this stage, or transfer to a refrigerator and chill thoroughly.

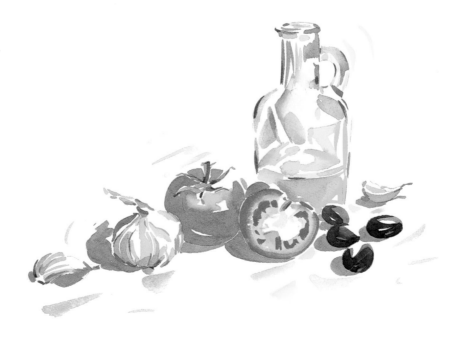

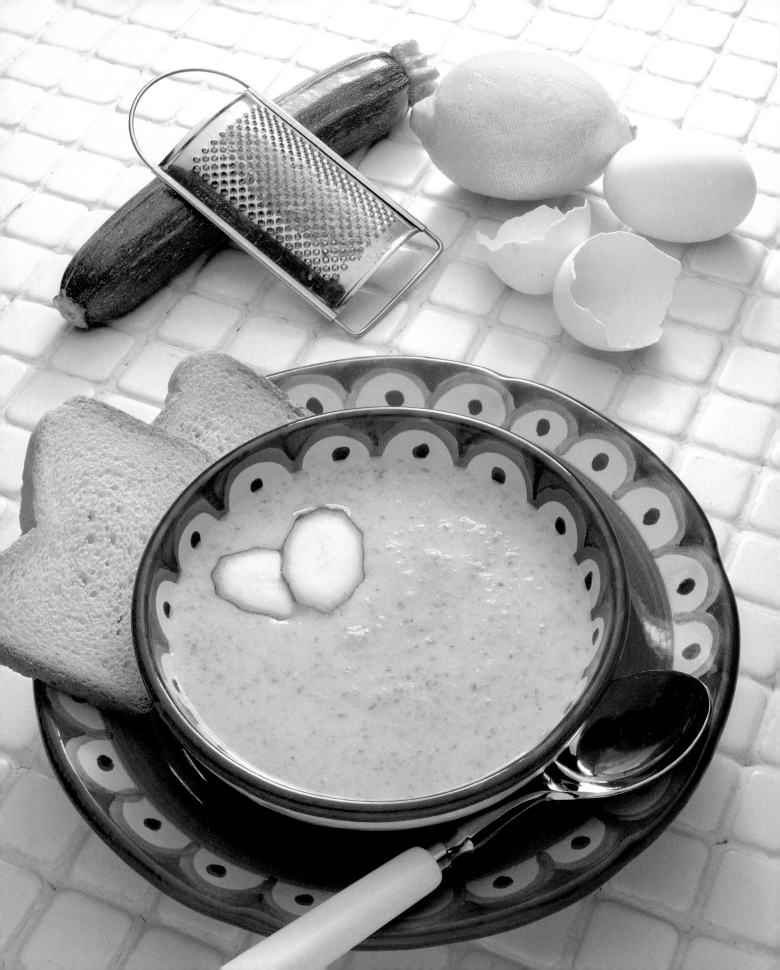

Casserole of Veal and Mushrooms

Preparation Time: 30 minutes **Cooking Time:** 1½ hours **Serves:** 6

Veal is a low fat meat and is delicious when served in this tomato and mushroom sauce.

Ingredients
1.5kg/3lbs lean pie veal
Salt and pepper
4 tbsps olive oil
2 shallots, finely chopped
½ clove garlic, crushed
6 tbsps dry white wine
280ml/½ pint strong brown stock

1 x 225g/8oz can tomatoes, drained
  and chopped
1 bouquet garni
2 strips lemon peel
120g/4oz small button mushrooms
2 tbsps fresh chopped parsley

Dice the meat into bite-sized pieces, using a sharp knife. Sprinkle the pieces of meat with salt and pepper, then allow to stand for about 30 minutes.

Heat half of the oil in a large frying pan, and cook the pieces of meat for 5-10 minutes, stirring them frequently until they are browned on all sides. Remove the meat from the pan and set it aside. Add the shallots and garlic to the oil and meat juices in the pan, lower the heat and cook until softened, but not coloured. Return the veal to the pan and mix well. Add the wine, stock, tomatoes, bouquet garni and lemon peel to the meat mixture, and bring to the boil. Transfer the veal to an ovenproof casserole. Cover with a tight fitting lid and bake in a pre-heated oven 160°C/325°F/Gas Mark 3 for about 1¼ hours, or until the meat is tender.

Heat the remaining oil in a clean frying pan, and gently stir in the mushrooms, cooking them for 2-3 minutes until they begin to soften, but are not properly cooked. After the casserole cooking time has finished, stir in the partially cooked mushrooms and continue cooking in the oven for a further 15 minutes. Sprinkle with the chopped parsley before serving.

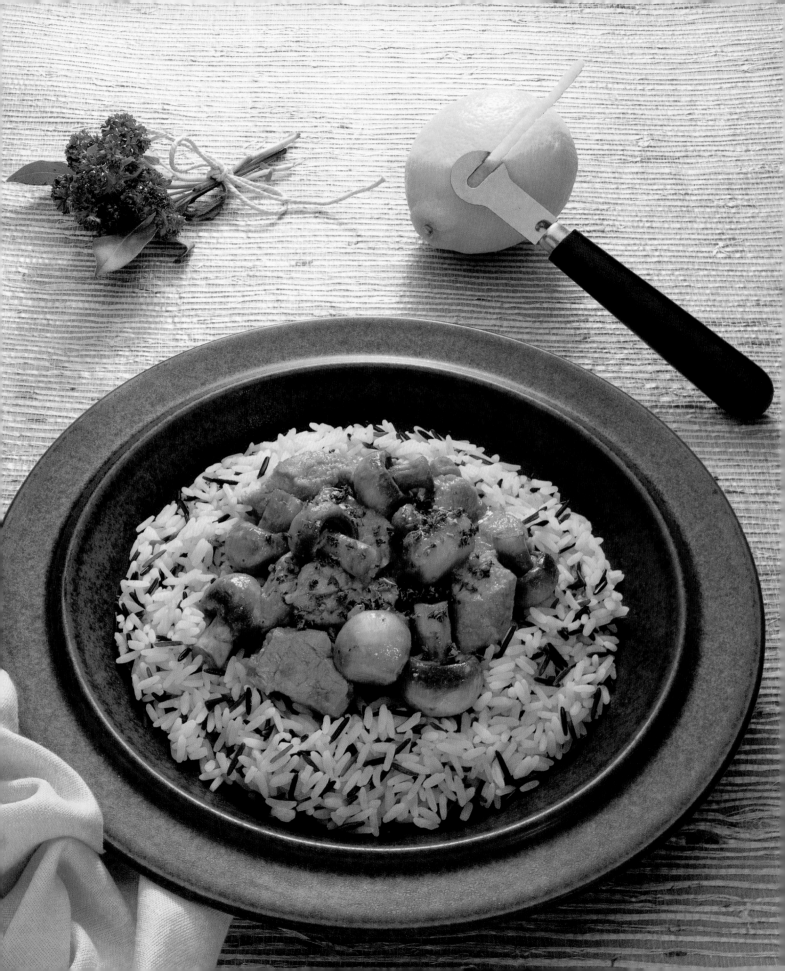

Ratatouille

Preparation Time: 20 minutes, plus 30 minutes standing time **Cooking Time:** 35 minutes **Serves:** 6

This delicious vegetable casserole from the south of France has become a great favourite the world over.

Ingredients

2 aubergines
4 tbsps olive oil
2 Spanish onions, thinly sliced
2 green or red peppers, seeded and roughly chopped
4 courgettes, thickly sliced

2 × 793g/1lb 12oz cans of tomatoes
1 large clove garlic, crushed
2 tsps chopped fresh basil
140ml/¼ pint dry white wine
Salt and pepper

Cut the aubergines in half lengthways, score each cut surface diagonally, using the point of a sharp knife and sprinkle them liberally with salt and allow to stand for 30 minutes to degorge. After this time, rinse them thoroughly, pat dry, and chop roughly.

Heat the oil in a large saucepan, and fry the onion slices for 5 minutes until they are soft and just beginning to brown. Stir in the peppers and courgettes, and cook gently for 5 minutes until they begin to soften. Remove all the vegetables from the pan and set them aside. Put the chopped aubergine into the saucepan with the vegetable juices. Cook gently until it begins to brown, then add all the other ingredients to the pan.

Add the tomatoes, garlic and basil to the saucepan along with the sautéed vegetables, mixing well to blend in evenly. Bring to the boil, then reduce the heat and simmer for 15 minutes, or until the liquid in the pan has been reduced and is thick. Add the wine to the pan, season to taste, and continue cooking for a further 15 minutes, before serving straight away, or chilling and serving cold.

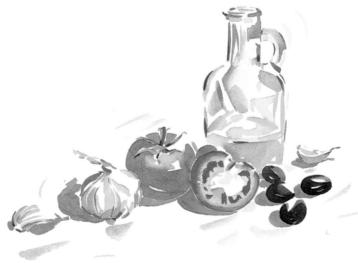

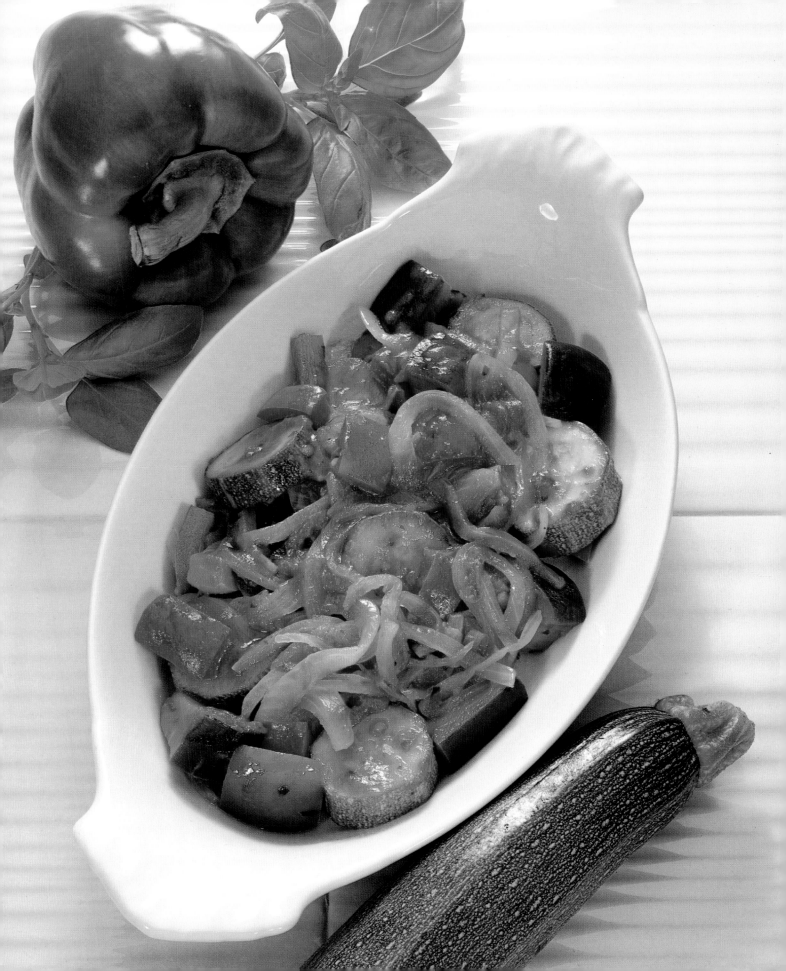

Sole Kebabs

Preparation Time: 30 minutes, plus marinating time
Cooking Time: 8 minutes **Serves:** 4

Fish is highly nutritious, economical to prepare, and makes an ideal contribution to a healthy diet.

Ingredients

8 fillets of sole
4 tbsps olive oil
1 clove garlic, crushed
Juice ½ lemon
Finely grated rind ½ lemon
Salt and pepper

3 drops Tabasco, or pepper sauce
3 courgettes, thinly sliced
1 green pepper, cut in 2.5cm/1-inch
  squares
Freshly chopped parsley for garnish

Using a sharp knife, carefully peel the skin from the backs of each sole fillet. Cut each sole fillet in half lengthways, and roll each slice up 'Swiss roll' fashion. Mix together the oil, garlic, lemon juice, rind, and seasonings in a small bowl. Put the rolls of fish into a shallow dish and pour over the lemon and oil marinade. Cover the dish and allow to stand in a cool place for at least 2 hours.

Carefully thread the marinated sole fillets onto kebab skewers, alternating these with pieces of the prepared vegetables. Brush each kebab with a little of the oil and lemon marinade. Arrange the kebabs on a grill pan and cook under a moderately hot grill for about 8 minutes, or cook outside on a barbecue, turning frequently to prevent them from burning, and brushing with the extra marinade to keep them moist. Arrange the kebabs on a serving dish, and sprinkle with the chopped parsley for garnish.

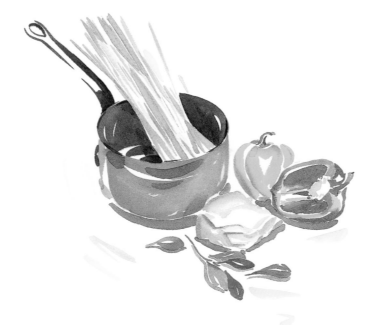

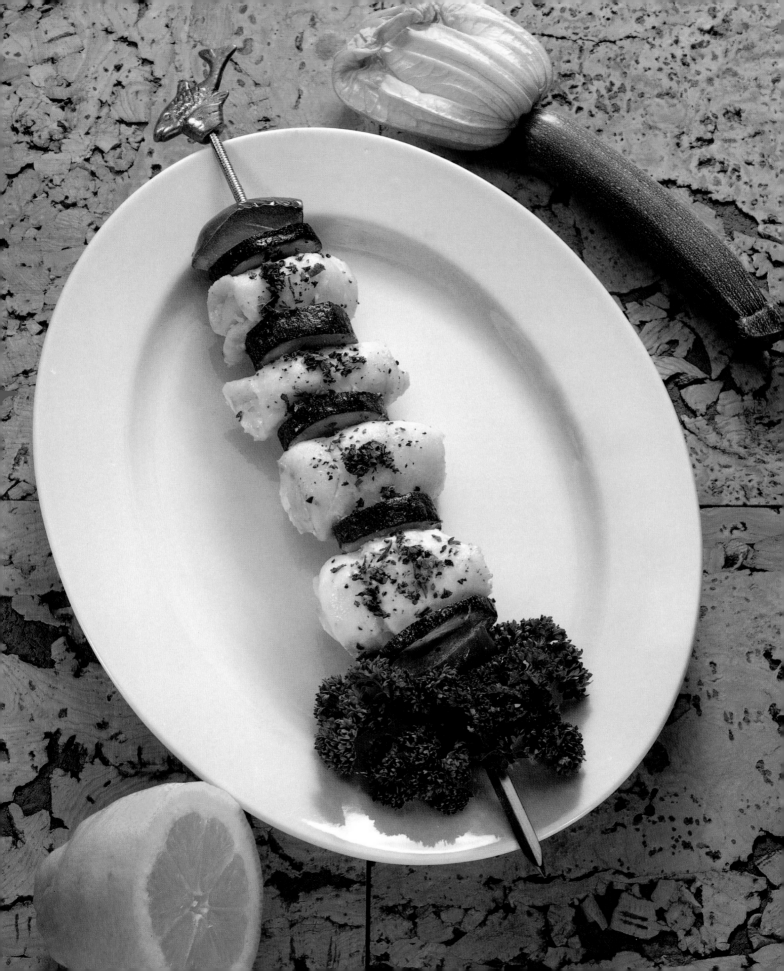

Salade Paysanne

Preparation Time: 20 minutes **Serves:** 6

This homely salad can be made with any selection of fresh vegetables you have to hand. So whether it's winter or summer, there's no excuse for not serving a delicious fresh salad.

Ingredients
8 lettuce leaves
4 spring onions, thinly sliced diagonally
½ cucumber, peeled, quartered, seeded and diced
3 carrots, thinly sliced, diagonally
6 large tomatoes, quartered
10 button mushrooms, thinly sliced
3 stems celery, thinly sliced
1 green pepper, seeded and chopped
15-20 tiny cauliflower florets
15-20 radishes, quartered

1 tbsp chopped watercress, or mustard and cress
2 sprigs fresh green coriander leaf, or chopped parsley

Dressing
2 tbsps cider vinegar
1 tbsp lemon juice
4 tbsps olive or vegetable oil
Pinch of mustard powder
Liquid sweetener to taste
Salt and pepper

Arrange the lettuce leaves on a serving dish, and pile the prepared salad vegetables on top. Whisk the dressing ingredients thoroughly using a fork, or balloon whisk, until the mixture becomes thick and cloudy.

Just before serving, spoon a little of the dressing over the salad and serve the remainder separately in a small jug.

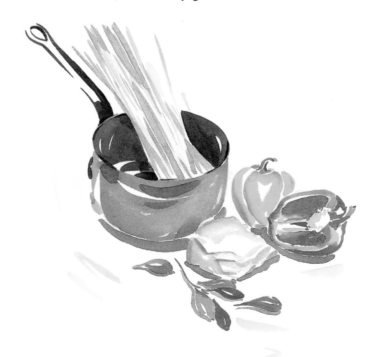

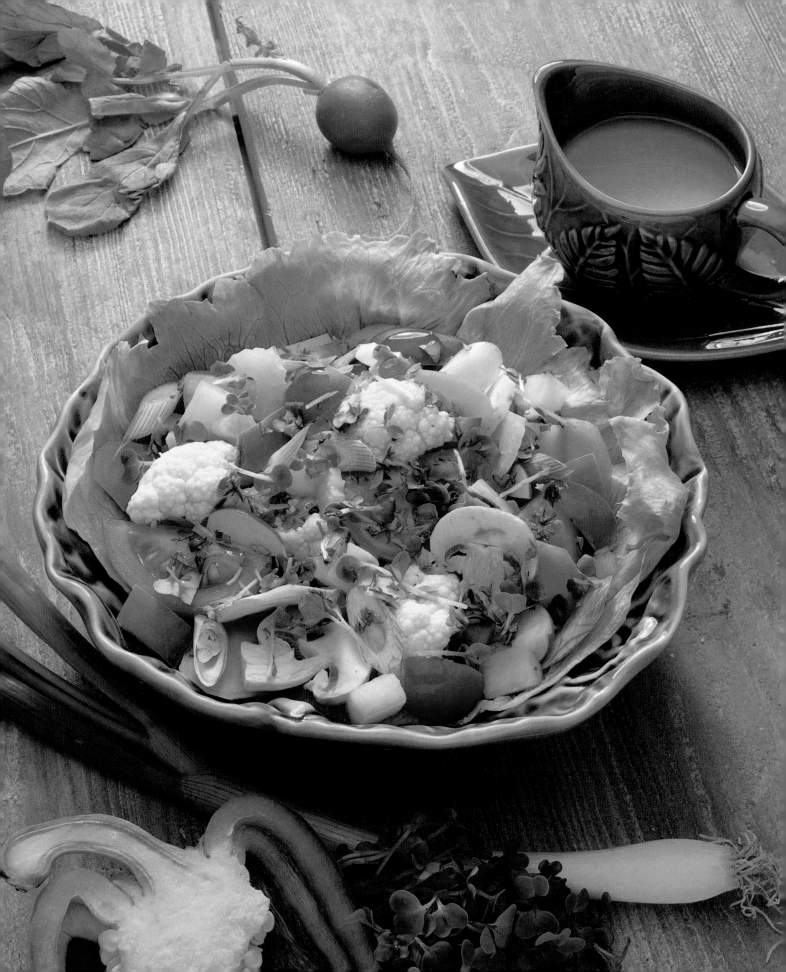

Kidneys with Mustard Sauce

Preparation Time: 25 minutes **Cooking Time:** 15 minutes **Serves:** 4

Lambs' kidneys have a wonderful delicate flavour, and when served with a delicious mustard sauce, make a quick and very flavoursome main course.

Ingredients
675g/1½lbs lambs' kidneys
4 tbsps vegetable oil
1-2 shallots, finely chopped
280ml/½ pint dry white wine

3 tbsps Dijon mustard
Salt, pepper and lemon juice, to taste
2 tbsps fresh chopped parsley

Cut the kidneys in half lengthways, and carefully snip out the core and tough tubes. Heat the oil in a large frying pan, and gently sauté the kidneys for about 10 minutes, stirring them frequently until they are light brown on all sides. Remove the kidneys from the pan and keep them warm.

Add the shallots to the sauté pan and cook for about 1 minute, stirring frequently until they soften, but do not brown. Add the wine and bring to the boil, stirring constantly and scraping the pan to remove any brown juices.

Allow the wine to boil rapidly for 3-4 minutes, until it has reduced by about two-thirds. Remove the pan from the heat. Using a balloon whisk or fork, mix the mustard into the reduced wine along with salt, pepper and lemon juice to taste, and half of the fresh chopped parsley.

Return the kidneys to the pan and cook over a low heat for 1-2 minutes, stirring all the time to heat the kidneys through evenly. Serve immediately, sprinkled with the remaining parsley.

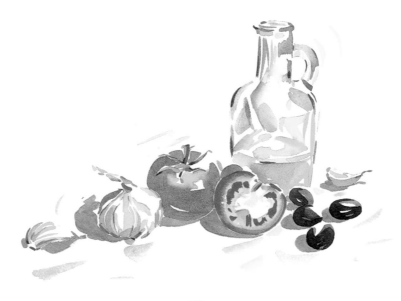

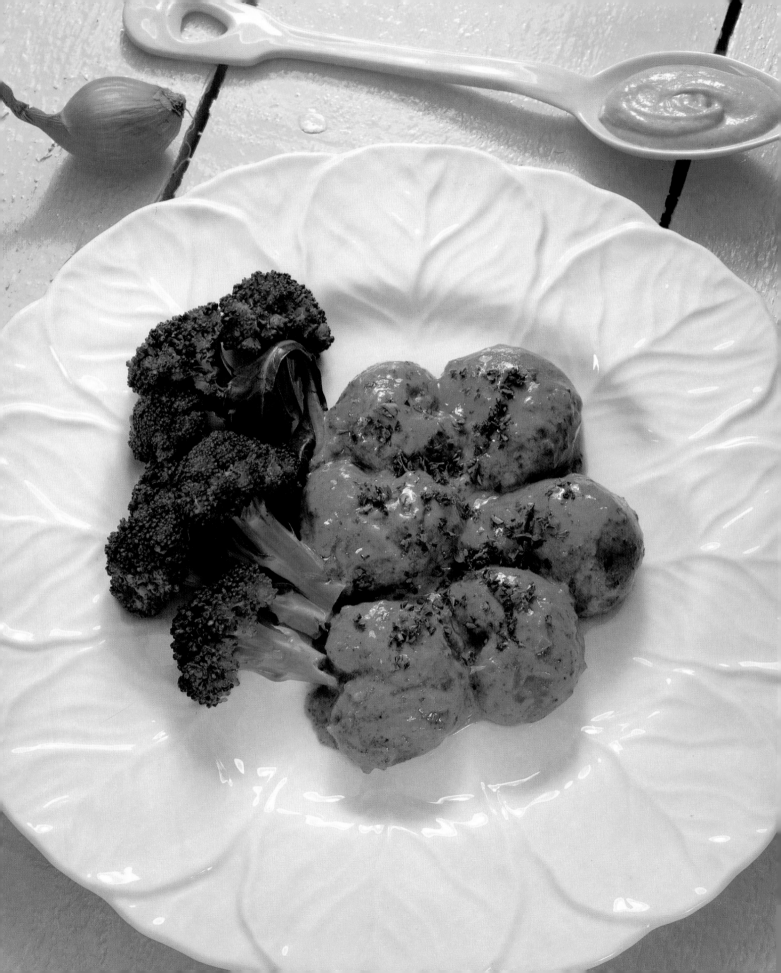

Lime Roasted Chicken

Preparation Time: 25 minutes, plus 4 hours marinating time **Cooking Time:** 40 minutes **Serves:** 4

This simply made, but unusual, main course is low in calories and high in tangy flavour.

Ingredients

4 chicken breast portions, each
   weighing about 225g/8oz
Salt and pepper
4 limes

2 tsps white wine vinegar
5 tbsps olive oil
2 tsps fresh chopped basil

Rub the chicken portions all over with salt and pepper. Place in a shallow ovenproof dish, and set aside. Carefully pare away thin strips of the rind from 2 of the limes, using a lemon parer. Cut these 2 limes in half and squeeze the juice. Add the lime juice to the vinegar and 4 tbsps of the olive oil in a small dish, along with the strips of rind, and mix well. Pour the oil and lime juice mixture over the chicken portions in the dish. Cover and refrigerate for about 4 hours or overnight.

Remove the covering from the dish in which the chicken is marinating, and baste the chicken well with the marinade mixture. Place into a preheated oven 190°C/375°F/Gas Mark 5 and cook for 30-35 minutes, or until the chicken is well roasted and tender.

In the meantime, peel away the rind and white pith from the remaining 2 limes. Cut the limes into thin slices using a sharp knife. Heat the remaining oil in a small frying pan and add the lime slices and basil. Cook quickly for 1 minute, or until the fragrance rises up from the basil and the limes just begin to soften. Serve the chicken portions on a serving platter, garnished with the fried lime slices and a little extra fresh basil, if desired.

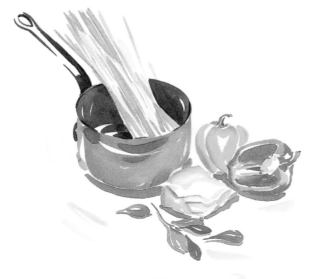

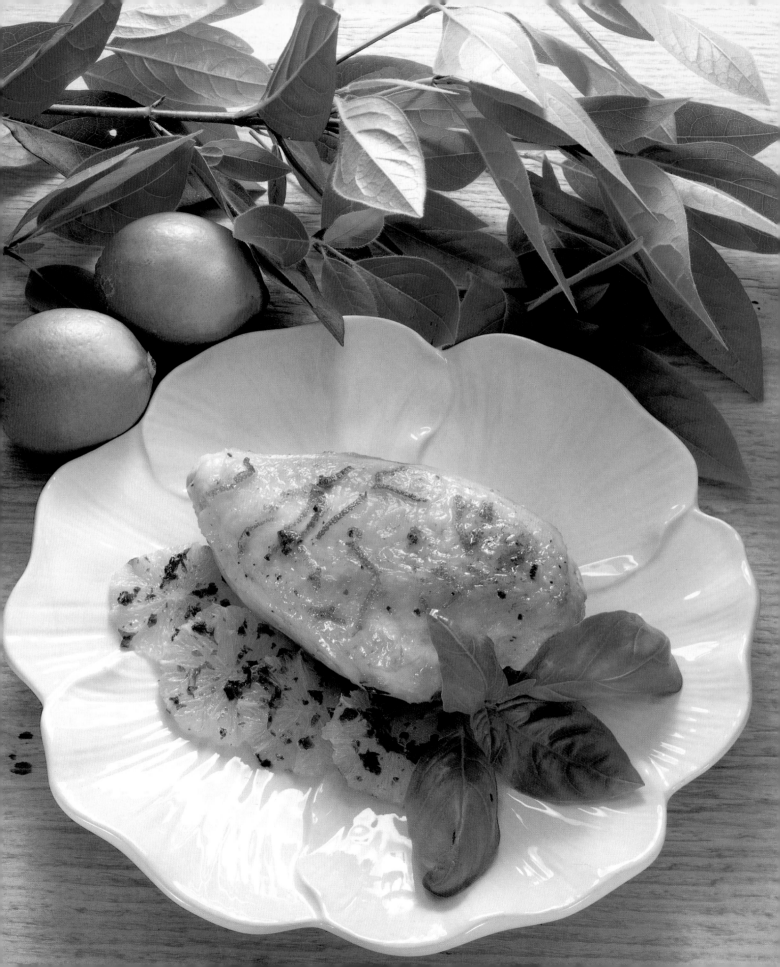

Aubergine Bake

Preparation Time: 30 minutes **Cooking Time:** 40 minutes **Serves:** 6

Aubergines are wonderfully filling vegetables with very few calories – the ideal ingredient in a calorie controlled diet.

Ingredients

2 large or 3 medium-sized
   aubergines
140ml/¼ pint malt vinegar
2 tbsps vegetable oil
2 large onions, sliced into rings
2 green chillies, seeded and finely
   chopped
1 × 425g/15oz can tomatoes,
   chopped
½ tsp chilli powder
1 clove garlic, crushed

½ tsp ground turmeric
8 tomatoes, sliced
280ml/½ pint natural unset yogurt
Salt and pepper
90g/3oz Cheddar cheese, finely
   grated

Cut the aubergines into 5mm/¼-inch thick slices. Arrange the slices in a shallow dish and sprinkle with 1 tsp salt. Pour over the malt vinegar, cover the dish and marinate for 30 minutes. Drain the aubergine well, discarding the marinade liquid.

Heat the vegetable oil in a frying pan and gently fry the onion rings until they are golden brown. Add the chillies, some salt to taste, chopped tomatoes, chilli powder, garlic and turmeric. Mix well and simmer for 5-7 minutes until thick and well blended.

Remove the sauce from the heat, cool slightly, and liquidize in a food processor until smooth. Arrange half of the aubergine slices in the base of a lightly greased shallow ovenproof dish. Spoon half of the tomato sauce over the aubergine slices. Cover the tomato sauce with the remaining aubergine, and then top this with the remaining tomato sauce and sliced tomatoes.

Mix together the yogurt, 1 tsp freshly ground black pepper and the Cheddar cheese. Pour this mixture over the tomato slices. Preheat an oven to 190°C/375°F/Gas Mark 5, and cook the aubergine bake for 20-30 minutes, or until the cheese topping bubbles and turns golden brown. Serve hot straight from the oven.

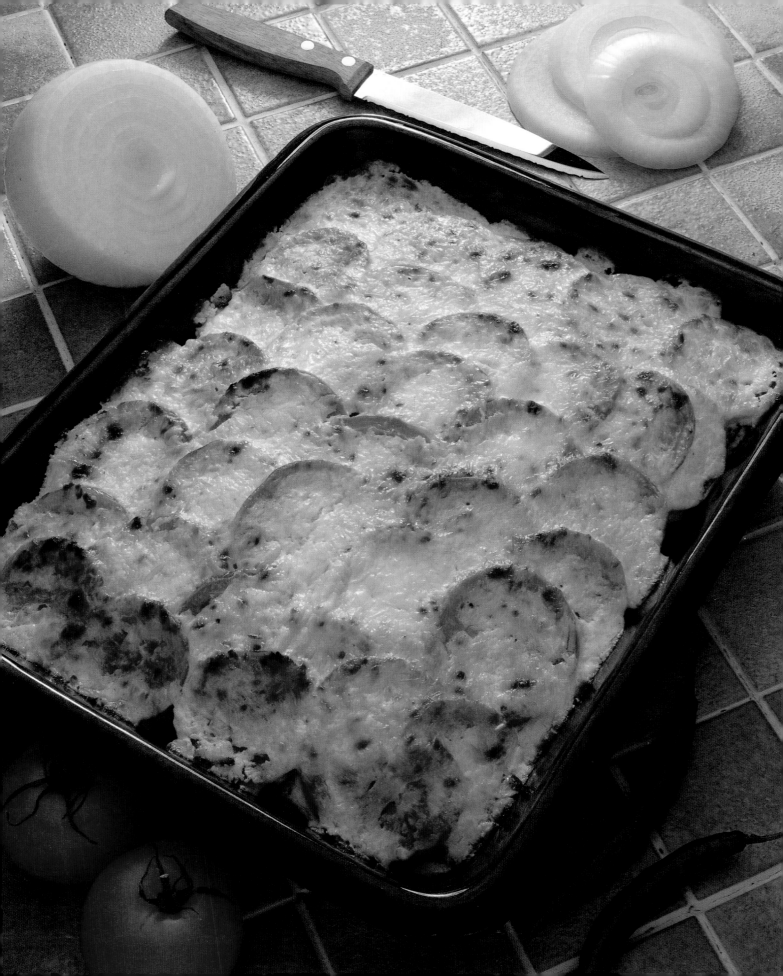

Vegetable Kebabs

Preparation Time: 30 minutes, plus 30 minutes marinating time
Cooking Time: 10 minutes **Serves:** 4

A colourful and flavoursome way to serve delicious fresh vegetables that can be grilled inside or barbecued outside.

Ingredients

1 large aubergine
1 large green pepper, seeded and cut
   in 2.5cm/1-inch pieces
4 courgettes, thickly sliced
12-14 cherry tomatoes, red or yellow
12-14 pickling onions, peeled

12-14 button mushrooms, rinsed

Marinade

4 tbsps olive oil
2 tbsps lemon juice
Salt and pepper

Cut the aubergine in half and dice it into 2.5cm/1-inch pieces. Put the aubergine pieces into a large bowl, and sprinkle liberally with salt. Stir well and allow to stand for 30 minutes to degorge. Rinse the aubergine pieces thoroughly in a colander under cold water, to remove all traces of salt.

Put all the prepared vegetables into a large bowl and pour in the marinade ingredients. Mix well to coat evenly, cover with plastic wrap and allow to stand for about 30 minutes, stirring the vegetables once or twice to ensure they remain evenly coated.

Thread the vegetables alternately onto skewers and arrange them on a grill pan. Brush the kebabs with the marinade and grill for 3-4 minutes, turning frequently and basting with the marinade until they are evenly browned. Serve piping hot.

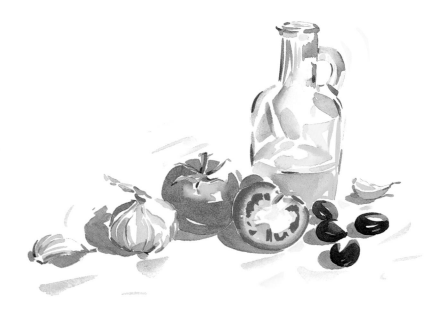

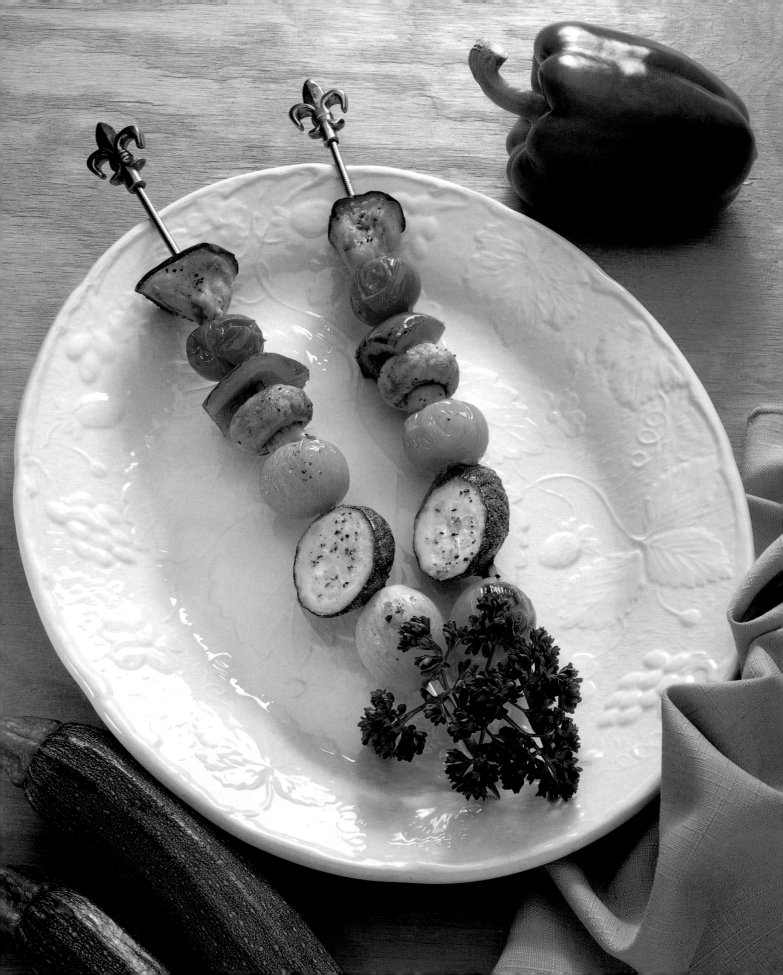

Liver with Onions

Preparation Time: 15 minutes **Cooking Time:** 10 minutes **Serves:** 4-6

This dish is simple to prepare, absolutely delicious and highly nutritious.

Ingredients

450g/1lb lambs' liver, thinly sliced
Salt and pepper
3 tbsps plain flour
3 tbsps vegetable oil

30g/1oz butter
450g/1lb onions, thinly sliced in rings
2 tbsps fresh chopped parsley

Trim away any large pipes or tubes from the liver using a pair of small scissors or a sharp knife. Mix the seasoning and the flour together on a plate and lay the slices of liver into the flour, turning them and pressing them gently to coat all over evenly.

Put the oil and the butter into a large frying pan. Heat gently until foaming. Add the onion rings and fry until just golden. Add the liver slices and fry for 3-5 minutes on each side until well cooked. Cooking time will depend on the thickness of each slice. Stir the parsley into the liver and onions and serve immediately on hot plates.

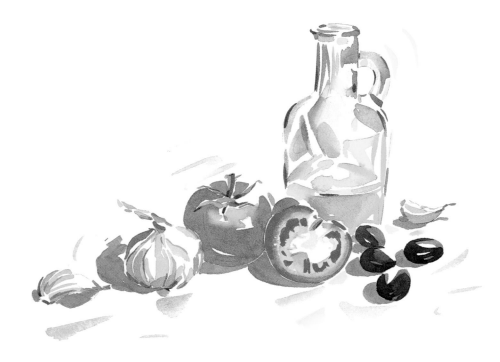

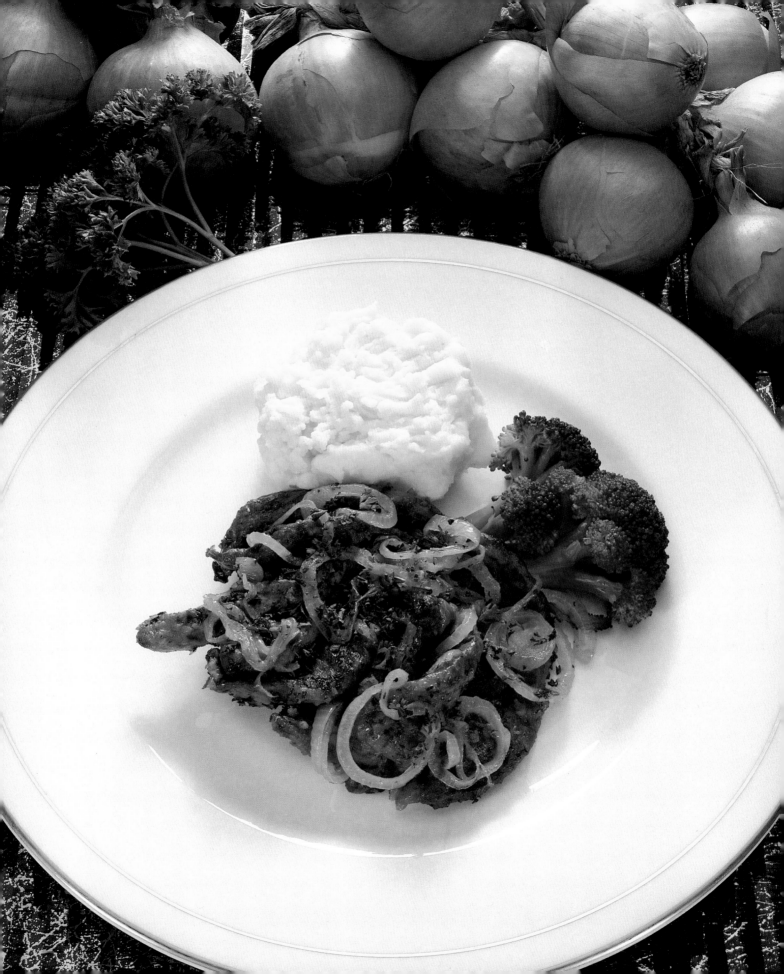

Tarragon Grilled Red Mullet

Preparation Time: 15 minutes, plus 30 minutes marinating time
Cooking Time: 10-16 minutes **Serves:** 4

Red mullet is a very decorative little fish that is now readily available at fishmongers and supermarkets.

Ingredients

4 large or 8 small red mullets, gutted, scaled, washed and dried
4 or 8 sprigs of fresh tarragon
4 tbsps vegetable oil
2 tbsps tarragon vinegar
Salt and pepper
1 egg
1 tsp Dijon mustard
120ml/4 fl oz sunflower oil
1 tbsp wine vinegar
1 tsp brandy
1 tbsp chopped fresh tarragon
1 tbsp chopped fresh parsley
1 tbsp double cream
Fresh tarragon to garnish

Rub the inside of each mullet with a teaspoonful of salt, scrubbing hard to remove any discoloured membranes inside. Rinse thoroughly. Place a sprig of fresh tarragon inside each fish. Using a sharp knife cut 2 diagonal slits on the side of each fish. Mix together the vegetable oil, tarragon vinegar and a little salt and pepper in a small bowl. Arrange the fish on a shallow dish and pour over the tarragon vinegar marinade, brushing some of the mixture into the cuts on the side of the fish. Refrigerate for 30 minutes.

Put the egg into a liquidizer along with the mustard and a little salt and pepper. Process for 2-3 seconds to mix. With the machine running, add the oil through the funnel in a thin steady stream. Continue blending the dressing until it is thick and creamy. Add the vinegar, brandy and herbs, and process for a further 30 seconds to mix well. Lightly whip the cream with a small whisk until it thickens. Fold the slightly thickened cream carefully into the oil and vinegar dressing. Pour into a serving dish and refrigerate until ready to use.

Arrange the fish on a grill pan and cook under a pre-heated hot grill for 5-8 minutes per side, depending on the size of the fish. Baste frequently with the marinade while cooking, then serve with the sauce and garnish with sprigs of fresh tarragon.

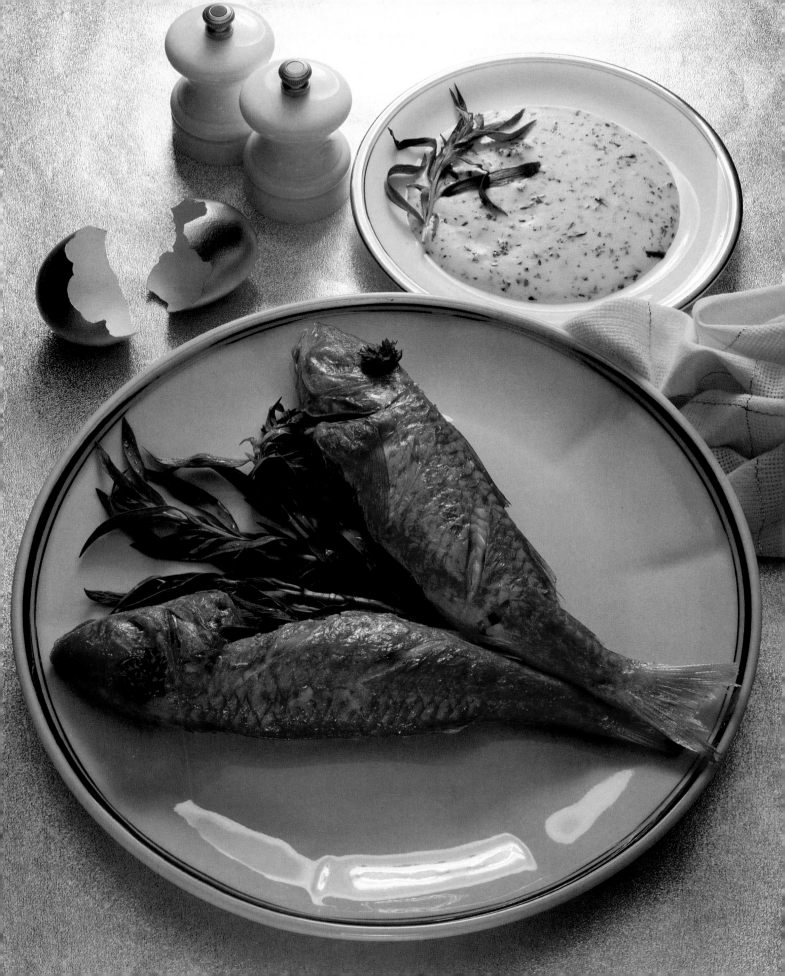

Beef with Pineapple and Peppers

Preparation Time: 30 minutes **Cooking Time:** 10 minutes **Serves:** 4

This delicious sweet and sour main course is Chinese in origin.

Ingredients

1 tbsp peanut oil
1 onion, roughly chopped
2 cloves garlic, crushed
2.5cm/1-inch piece fresh ginger, peeled and thinly sliced
450g/1lb fillet or rump steak, cut in thin strips
1 green pepper, seeded and thinly sliced
1 red pepper, seeded and thinly sliced
1 small pineapple, peeled, sliced, cored and chopped
1 tsp sesame oil
2 tbsps light soy sauce
1 tbsp dark soy sauce
1 tsp sugar
1 tbsp brown sauce
4 tbsps water
Salt and pepper

Heat the peanut oil in a wok or large frying pan, and gently fry the onion, garlic and ginger, stirring continuously until the onion has softened slightly. Add the strips of beef and the strips of pepper, and continue stir-frying for 3 minutes.

Add the pineapple and stir-fry again for 2 minutes.

Remove the meat, vegetables and fruit from the wok, and put on a plate. Set aside.

Stir the sesame oil into the juices in the wok and add the soy sauces, sugar, brown sauce and water. Simmer rapidly for 30 seconds to reduce and thicken.

Stir the fruit, vegetables and beef back into the sauce. Season, heat through and serve immediately.

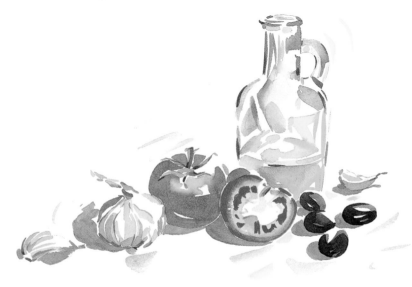

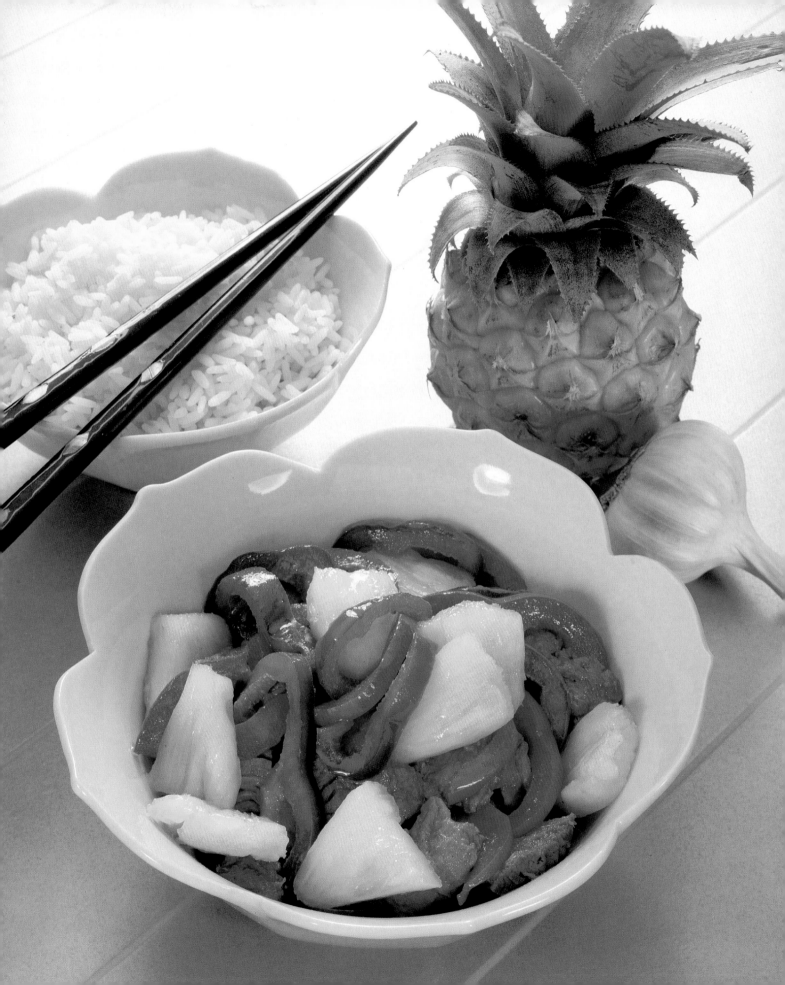

Cheese Salad

Preparation Time: 10-12 minutes **Serves:** 4

This cheese salad is Greek in origin, and is ideal as a starter as well as being substantial enough to serve as a light lunch.

Ingredients

½ small head of endive, washed and torn into bite-sized pieces
½ small iceberg lettuce, washed and torn into bite-sized pieces
1 small cucumber, thinly sliced
4 large tomatoes, sliced
8-10 pitted green or black olives, halved
1 medium-sized Spanish or red onion, sliced

120g/4oz feta cheese, cut in 1.25cm/ ½-inch cubes

Dressing

5 tbsps olive oil
2 tbsps red wine vinegar
1 tsp chopped fresh oregano
Salt and pepper
½ tsp German mustard

Put the endive, lettuce, cucumber, tomatoes, olives and onion into a serving bowl and toss them together until well mixed. Sprinkle feta cubes over the salad in the serving bowl.

Put the dressing ingredients into a small bowl and whisk together using a fork or small whisk. Pour the dressing over the salad and serve immediately.

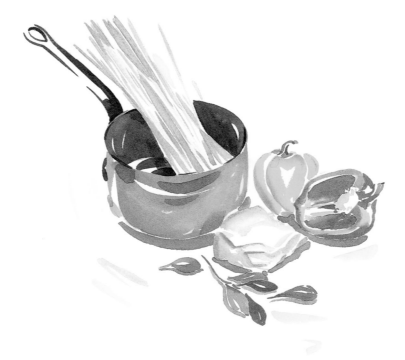

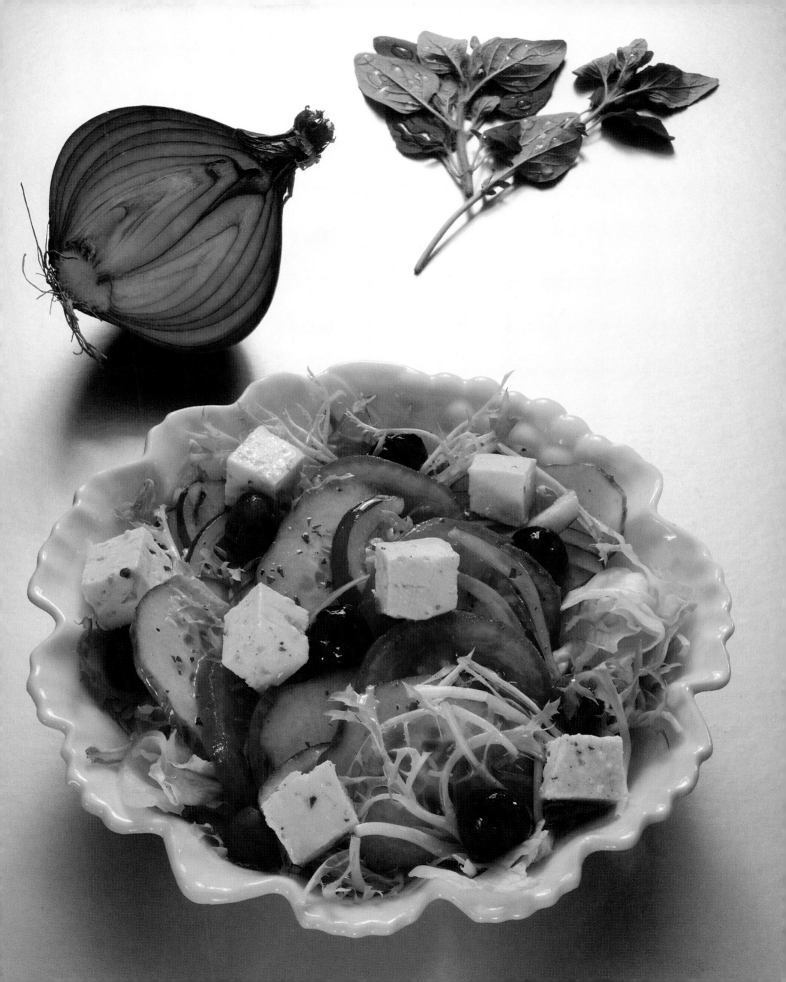

Dolmas

Preparation Time: 30 minutes **Cooking Time:** 40 minutes **Serves:** 6

Delicious individual parcels of rice, herbs, nuts and fruit, make a very different low calorie lunch or supper dish.

Ingredients

12 large cabbage leaves, washed
180g/6oz long grain rice
8 spring onions, thinly sliced
   diagonally
1 tbsp fresh chopped basil
1 tbsp fresh chopped mint
1 tbsp fresh chopped parsley

60g/2oz pine nuts
60g/2oz currants
Salt and pepper
4 tbsps olive oil
Juice 1 lemon
140ml/¼ pint unset natural yogurt
120g/4oz cucumber

Using a sharp knife trim away any tough stems from the cabbage leaves. Put the leaves into boiling water for about 30 seconds. Remove them using a slotted spoon and drain thoroughly before laying them out flat on a work surface. Put the rice into a saucepan along with enough boiling water to just cover. Cook for 15-20 minutes, or until the rice is soft and the liquid almost completely absorbed. Rinse the rice in cold water to remove any starchiness. Put the rice and the chopped onions into a large bowl along with all the remaining ingredients, except 2 tbsps olive oil, the yogurt and cucumber. Mix the rice mixture thoroughly to blend evenly.

Place about 2 tbsps of the rice filling onto each blanched cabbage leaf, pressing it gently into a sausage shape. Fold the sides of the leaves over to partially cover the stuffing, and then roll up, Swiss roll fashion, to completely envelop the filling. Place the rolls seam side down in a large baking dish. Brush with the remaining olive oil. Pour hot water around the cabbage leaves until it comes about halfway up their sides. Cover the baking dish with aluminium foil, pressing it gently onto the surface of the leaves to keep them in place. Bake in a preheated oven 190°C/375°F/Gas Mark 5 for 30-40 minutes.

Peel the cucumber and cut it lengthways into quarters. Remove the pips and discard. Chop the cucumber flesh and half of the peel into very small pieces. Mix the chopped cucumber into the yogurt and chill until required. Drain the dolmas from the cooking liquid and arrange on a serving plate with a little of the cucumber sauce spooned over.

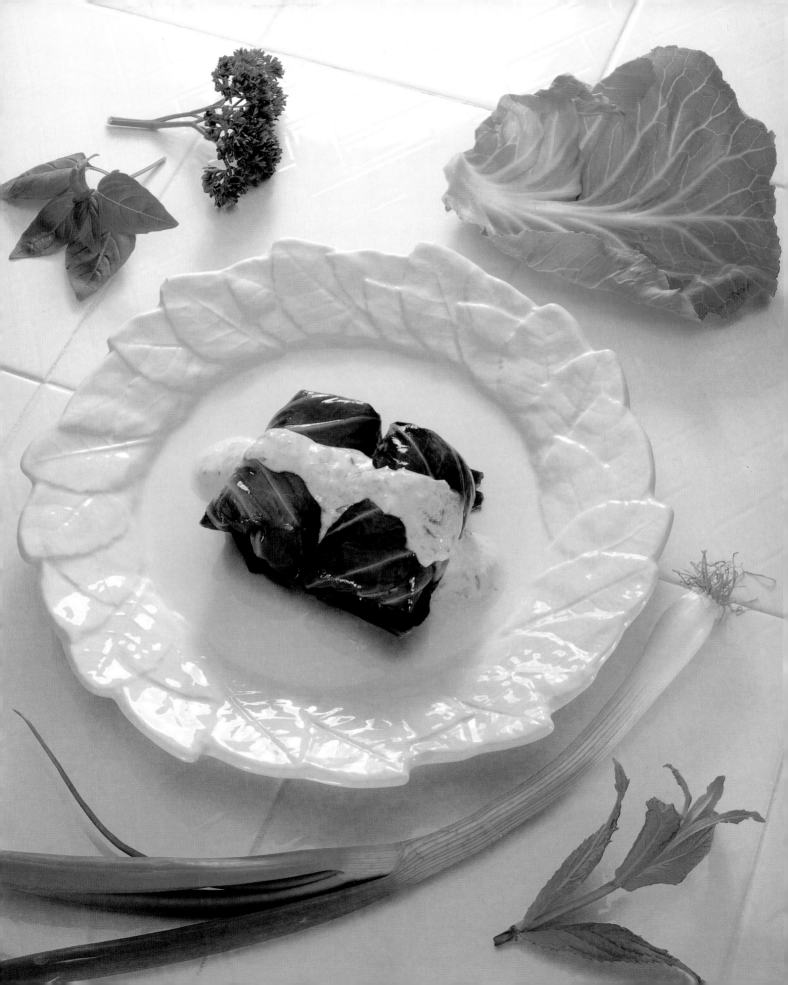

Swedish Herrings

Preparation Time: 10 minutes **Cooking Time:** 12-15 minutes **Serves:** 4

The Swedes adore the flavour of fresh dill and mild mustard. This combination is all that is required to bring out the full flavour of fresh herring.

Ingredients

4 tbsps fresh chopped dill
90ml/6 tbsps mild Swedish mustard
2 tbsps lemon juice or white wine
4-8 fresh herrings, cleaned, but
    heads and tails left on

2 tbsps unsalted butter, melted
Freshly ground black pepper
Lemon wedges and whole sprigs of
    fresh dill, to garnish

Put the dill, mustard and lemon juice or white wine into a small bowl and mix together thoroughly. Using a sharp knife, cut three shallow slits through the skin on both sides of each fish. Spread half of the mustard mixture over one side of each fish, pushing some of the mixture into each cut. Drizzle a little of the melted butter over the fish and grill under a preheated hot grill for 5-6 minutes.

Using a fish slice, carefully turn each fish over, and spread with the remaining dill and mustard mixture. Drizzle over the remaining butter and grill for a further 5-6 minutes, or until the fish is thoroughly cooked. Sprinkle the fish with black pepper and serve garnished with the dill sprigs and lemon wedges.

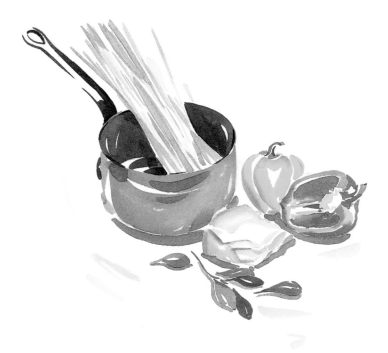

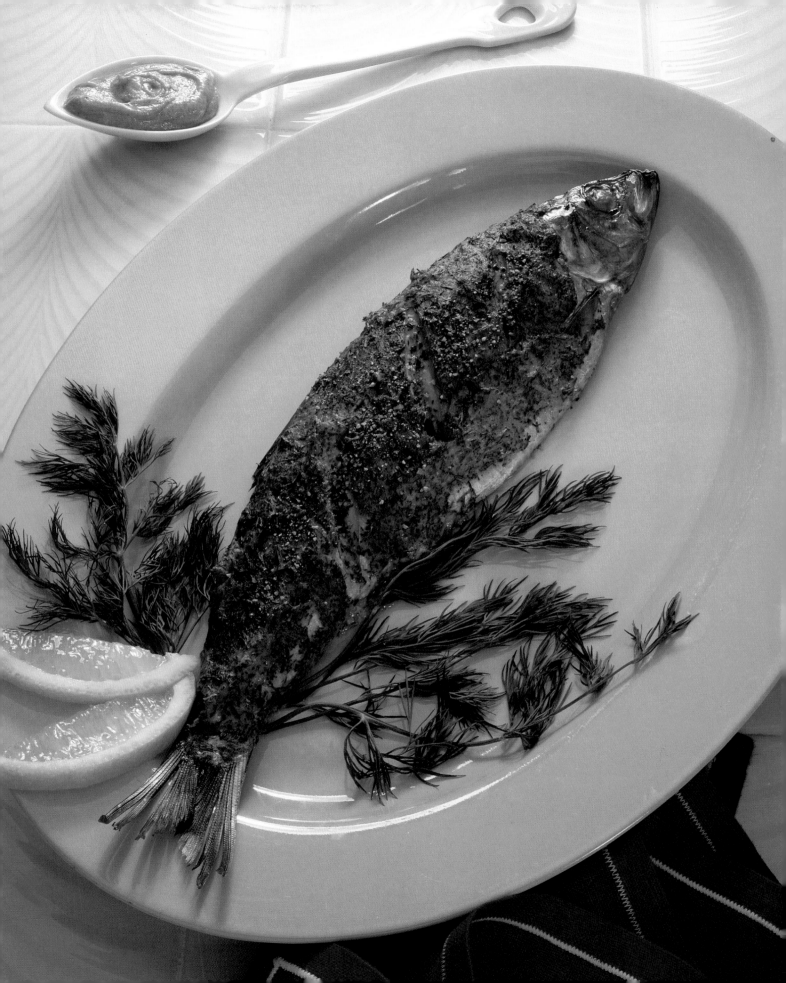

Ham and Green Pepper Omelette

Preparation Time: 15 minutes **Cooking Time:** 5 minutes **Makes:** 1

Use 'tendersweet' ham in this recipe to keep the salt content as low as possible.

Ingredients
3 eggs
2 tbsps milk
Freshly ground black pepper
1 tbsp vegetable oil

30g/1oz chopped green pepper
2 tomatoes, peeled, seeded and
 roughly chopped
60g/2oz lean ham, cut into small dice

Break the eggs into the bowl and beat in the milk and pepper. Heat the oil in an omelette pan and fry the green pepper until it is just soft. Stir in the tomatoes and the ham. Heat through for 1 minute. Pour the egg mixture into the frying pan over the vegetables. Stir the mixture briskly with a wooden spoon, until it begins to cook. As the egg begins to set, lift it slightly and tilt the pan to allow the uncooked egg underneath. When the egg on top is still slightly creamy, fold the omelette in half and slip it onto a serving plate. Serve immediately.

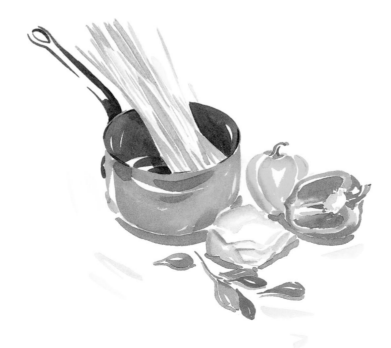

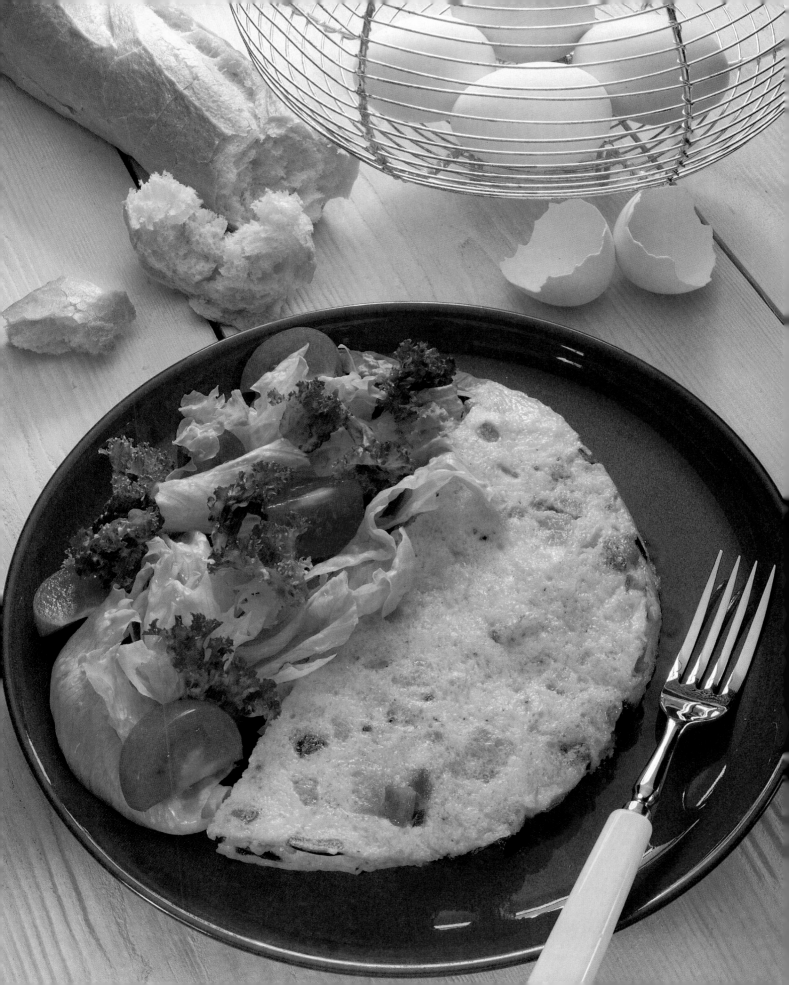

Turkey Kebabs

Preparation Time: 20 minutes, plus overnight marinating
Cooking Time: 30 minutes **Serves:** 6

For this low fat dish, use the ready-prepared turkey joints which are now easily available from supermarkets or butchers.

Ingredients

1.5kg/3lbs lean turkey meat

120g/4oz lean back bacon, rind removed
Whole sage leaves

Marinade
2 tsps fresh chopped sage
1 sprig rosemary, chopped
Juice 1 lemon
2 tbsps olive oil
Salt and pepper

Remove any bone from the turkey and cut the meat into even-sized cubes. Put the marinade ingredients into a large bowl and stir in the turkey meat, mixing well to coat evenly. Cover and leave in the refrigerator overnight.

Cut the bacon strips into half lengthways and then again crosswise. Wrap these pieces around as many of the cubes of marinated turkey meat as possible. Thread the turkey and bacon rolls alternately with the sage leaves and any unwrapped turkey cubes onto kebab skewers. Heat the grill to moderate, and cook the kebabs under the heat for 25-30 minutes, turning frequently and basting with the marinade. Serve immediately.

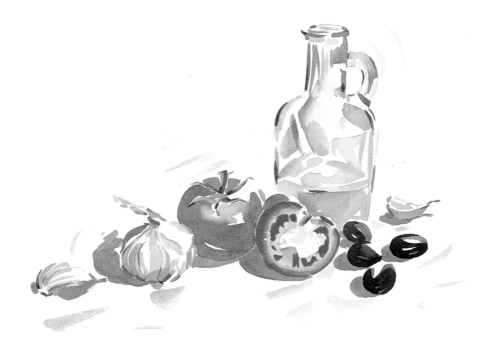

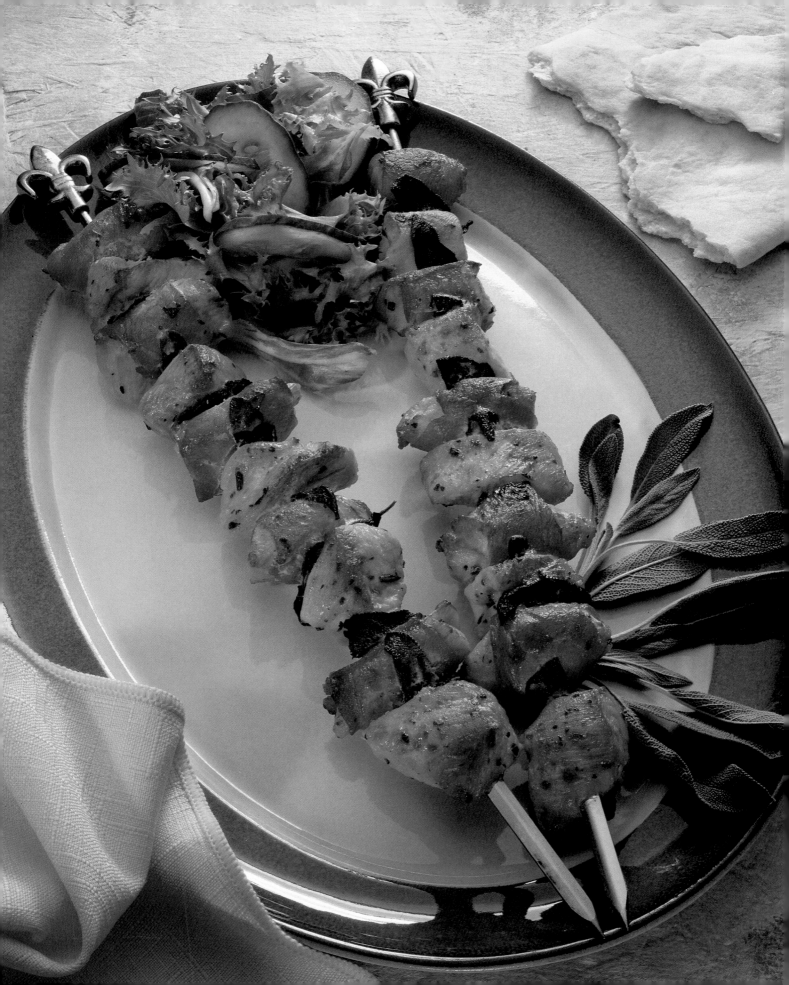

Chicken Liver Stir-Fry

Preparation Time: 25 minutes **Cooking Time:** 5-6 minutes **Serves:** 4

Chicken livers are very low in fat and high in flavour. They also require very little cooking so are perfect for stir-fry recipes.

Ingredients

3 tbsps sesame oil
60g/2oz split blanched almonds
1 clove garlic, peeled
450g/1lb chicken livers, trimmed and
  cubed
60g/2oz mange tout peas, trimmed

8-10 Chinese leaves, shredded
2 tsps cornflour
1 tbsp cold water
2 tbsps soy sauce
140ml/¼ pint chicken or vegetable
  stock

Heat a wok and pour in the oil. When the oil is hot, reduce the heat and stir-fry the almonds until they are pale golden brown. Remove the almonds, draining any oil back into the wok, and set them aside on absorbent kitchen paper. Add the garlic clove to the wok and cook for 1-2 minutes to flavour the oil only. Remove the clove of garlic and discard. Stir the chicken livers into the flavoured oil and cook for 2-3 minutes, stirring frequently to brown evenly. Remove the chicken livers from the wok and set them aside. Add the mange tout peas to the hot oil and stir-fry for 1 minute. Then stir in the Chinese leaves and cook for 1 minute further. Remove the vegetables and set aside.

  Mix together the cornflour and water, then blend in the soy sauce and stock. Pour the cornflour mixture into the wok and bring to the boil, stirring until the sauce has thickened and cleared. Return all other ingredients to the wok and heat through for 1 minute. Serve immediately.

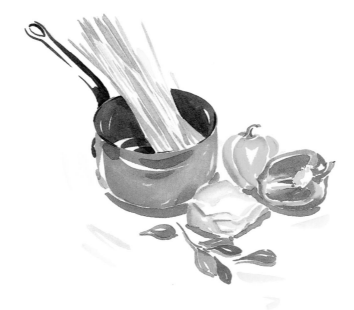

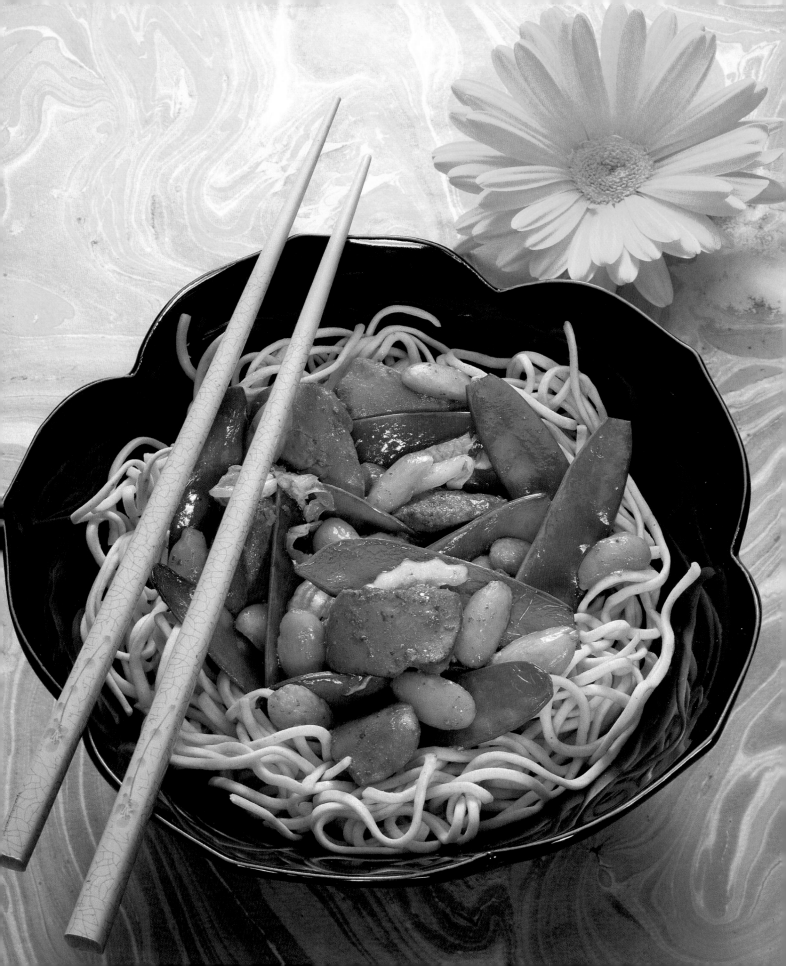

Summer Pasta Salad

Preparation Time: 40 minutes **Cooking Time:** 30 minutes Serves: 4

Lightly cooked summer vegetables and wholemeal pasta are combined to create this delicious wholesome salad.

Ingredients

1 aubergine
4 tbsps olive oil
1 medium-sized onion, finely
　chopped
1 courgette, sliced thinly
1 red pepper, cut in thin strips
1 green pepper, cut in thin strips

2 large tomatoes, skinned, seeded
　and sliced
1 clove garlic, crushed
Salt and pepper
225g/8oz wholemeal pasta spirals
1 tbsp vinegar
½ tsp dry English mustard

Cut the aubergine into 1cm/½-inch slices. Sprinkle the slices liberally with salt and allow to stand for 30 minutes. Thoroughly rinse the salt from the aubergine slices and pat them dry on absorbent kitchen paper. Roughly chop the slices.

Put 2 tbsps of the olive oil in a frying pan and stir in the onion. Fry gently until it is transparent, but not coloured. Add the chopped aubergine, courgette, peppers, tomatoes and garlic to the cooked onion and fry very gently for 20 minutes, or until just soft. Season with salt and pepper and allow to cool.

Put the pasta spirals in a large saucepan and cover with boiling water. Sprinkle in a little salt and simmer for 10 minutes or until tender but still firm. Rinse the pasta in cold water and drain very well.

Whisk together the remaining olive oil, the vinegar and mustard in a small bowl. Season with salt and pepper. Put the pasta and cooled vegetables into a serving dish and pour over the dressing, tossing the ingredients together to coat them evenly. Serve well chilled.

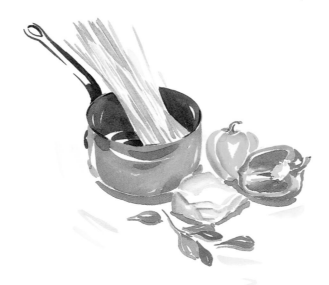

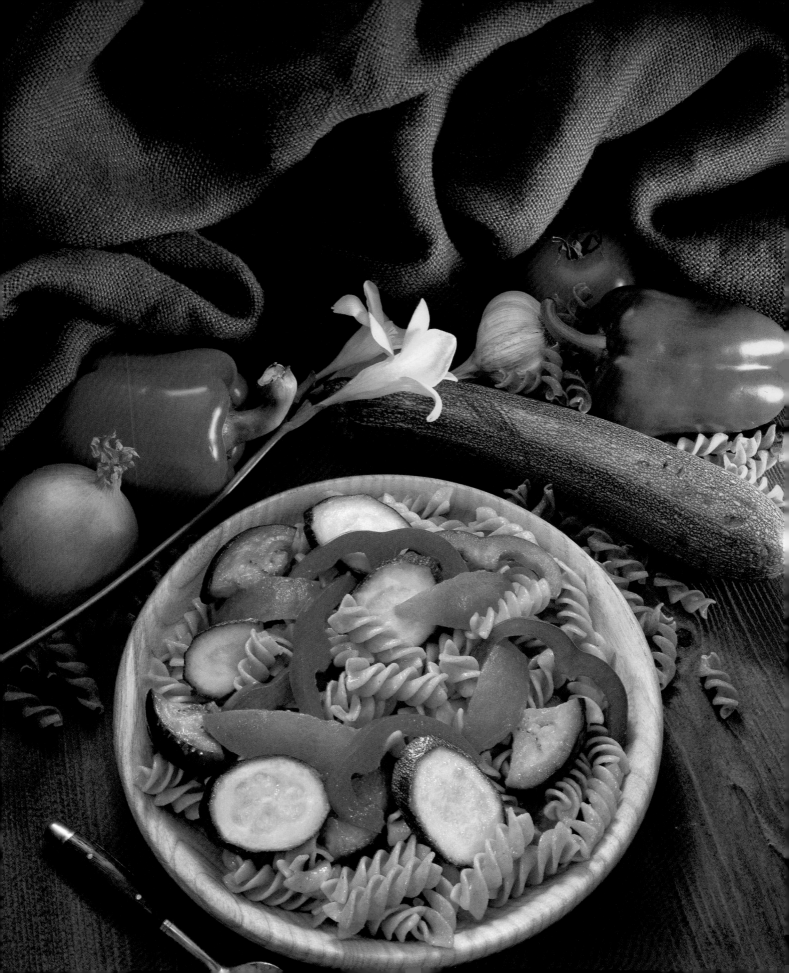

Andalusian Aubergines

Preparation Time: 40 minutes **Cooking Time:** 50 minutes **Serves:** 4

This delicious aubergine dish is highly reminiscent of Andalucia in Spain where tomatoes, rice and tuna fish are very popular ingredients.

Ingredients

4 small aubergines
3 tbsps olive oil
1 small onion, finely chopped
1 clove garlic, crushed
Freshly ground black pepper
120g/4oz cooked whole grain rice
1 x 200g/7oz can tuna in oil, drained
and fish coarsely flaked

1 tbsp mayonnaise
1 tsp curry powder
4 fresh tomatoes, skinned, seeded
and chopped
1 tbsp coarsely chopped parsley

Cut the aubergines in half lengthways. Score the cut surfaces lightly with a sharp knife at regular intervals. Brush the scored surface lightly with 1 tbsp of the olive oil and place the aubergines on a greased baking sheet. Bake the aubergines in a preheated oven 190°C/375°F/Gas Mark 5 for 15 minutes, or until beginning to soften. Cool the aubergines slightly, then carefully scoop the centre flesh from each half. Take care that you do not break the skin at this stage.

Fry the chopped onion gently in the remaining olive oil for 3 minutes, or until it is just transparent. Add the garlic and the aubergine flesh, and fry for a further 2 minutes. Season to taste with pepper. Add the rice, flaked tuna, mayonnaise, curry powder, tomatoes, parsley and more black pepper to the aubergine mixture, and mix together well.

Pile equal amounts of this rice and tuna filling into the aubergine shells. Return the filled aubergines to the ovenproof baking dish. Brush with olive oil, and bake in the oven for a further 25 minutes. Serve piping hot.

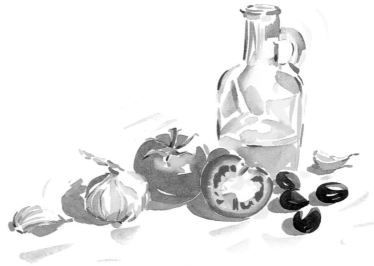

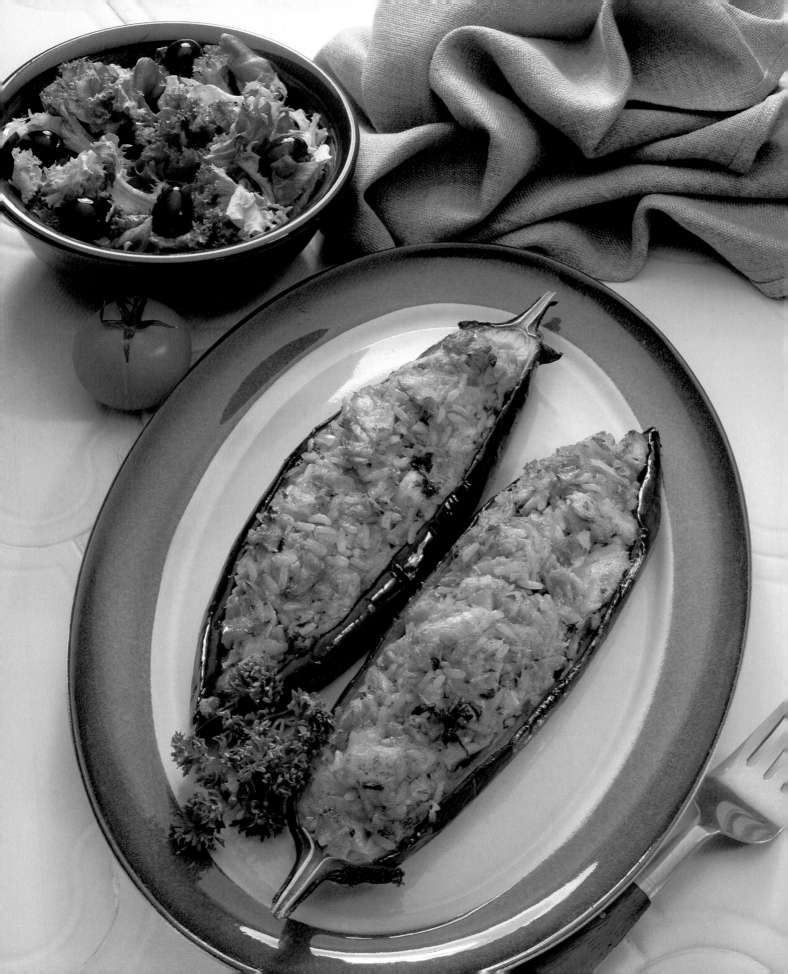

Chicken with 'Burnt' Peppers and Coriander

Preparation Time: 30 minutes **Cooking Time:** 1 hour 30 minutes **Serves:** 4

'Burning' peppers is a technique for removing the skins which also imparts a delicious flavour to this favourite vegetable.

Ingredients

2 red peppers, halved and seeded
1 green pepper, halved and seeded
4 tbsps vegetable oil, for brushing
1 tbsp olive oil
2 tsps paprika
¼ tsp ground cumin
Pinch cayenne pepper
2 cloves garlic, crushed
450g/1lb canned tomatoes, drained and chopped
3 tbsps fresh chopped coriander
3 tbsps fresh chopped parsley
Salt
4 large chicken breasts, boned
1 large onion, sliced
60g/2oz flaked almonds

Put the peppers, cut side down, on a flat surface and gently press them with the palm of your hand to flatten them out. Brush the skin side with 2 tbsps of the vegetable oil and cook them under a hot grill until the skin chars and splits. Wrap the peppers in a clean towel for 10 minutes to cool. Unwrap the peppers and carefully peel off the charred skin. Chop the pepper flesh into thin strips.

Heat the olive oil in a frying pan and gently fry the paprika, cumin, cayenne pepper and garlic for 2 minutes, stirring to prevent the garlic from browning. Stir in the tomatoes, coriander, parsley and season with a little salt. Simmer for 15-20 minutes, or until thick. Set aside.

Heat the remaining vegetable oil in a large casserole and sauté the chicken breasts, turning them frequently until they are golden brown on both sides. Remove the chicken and set aside. Gently fry the onions in the oil for about 5 minutes, or until softened but not overcooked. Return the chicken to the casserole with the onions and pour on about 280ml/½ pint of water. Bring to the boil, cover the casserole, and simmer for about 30 minutes, turning the chicken occasionally to prevent it from burning. Remove the chicken from the casserole and boil the remaining liquid rapidly to reduce to about 90ml/3 fl oz of stock. Add the peppers and the tomato sauce to the chicken stock and stir well. Return the chicken to the casserole, cover and simmer very gently for a further 30 minutes, or until the chicken is tender. Arrange the chicken on a serving dish with a little of the sauce spooned over. Sprinkle with flaked almonds and serve any remaining sauce separately.

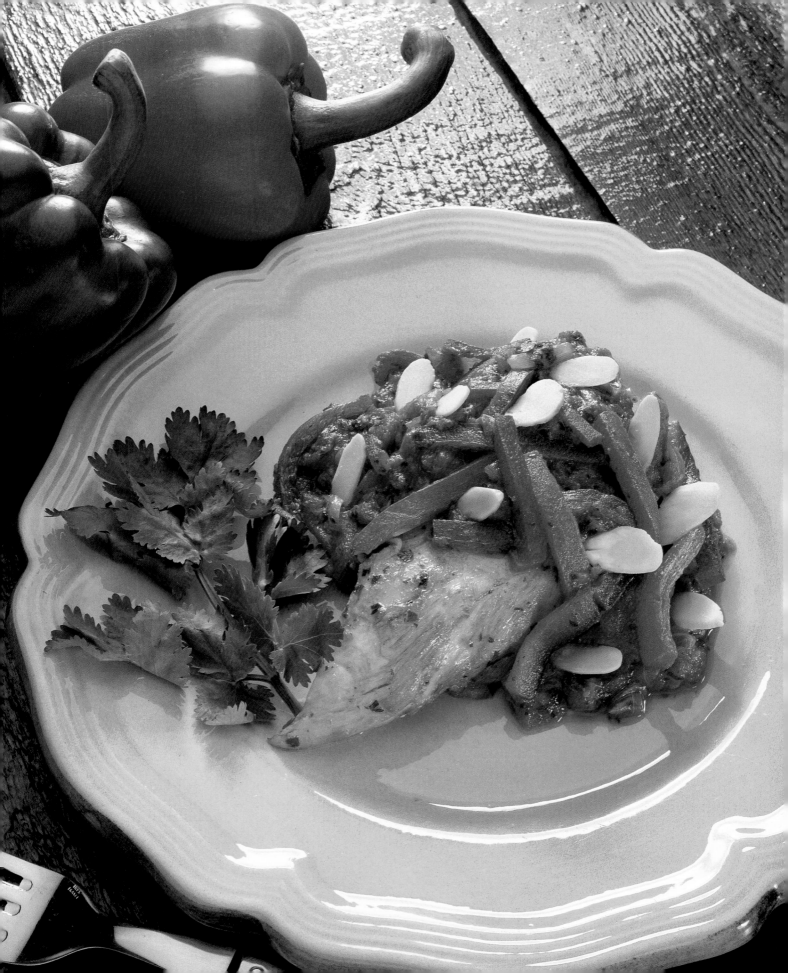

Honey and Apple Tart

Preparation Time: 45 minutes **Cooking Time:** 40 minutes **Serves:** 6

This delicious apple flan is wonderful served either hot or cold.

Ingredients

90g/3oz wholemeal flour
90g/3oz plain white flour
90g/3oz unsalted butter
1 egg yolk
3 tbsps cold water
280ml/½ pint unsweetened apple
   purée

1 tbsp honey
2 egg yolks
2 tbsps ground almonds
3 large eating apples, quartered,
   cored and thinly sliced
Little pale soft brown sugar
3 tbsps clear honey, warmed to glaze

Put the flours into a large bowl. Cut the butter into small pieces and rub these into the flour until the mixture resembles fine breadcrumbs. Beat the egg yolk and 2 tbsps of the water together. Stir this into the dry ingredients, mixing to a firm soft dough and adding a little extra water if necessary. Roll the dough on a lightly floured surface and line a 22.5cm/9-inch loose-bottom, fluted flan ring. Pinch up the edges well and prick the base to prevent it from rising during cooking.

Mix the apple purée with the honey, egg yolks and ground almonds, stirring well to blend thoroughly. Spread this apple mixture evenly over the base of the pastry case. Arrange the apple slices, overlapping slightly, in circles, on the top of the apple and almond filling. Sprinkle the top of the flan lightly with a little soft brown sugar, and bake in a preheated oven 190°C/375°F/Gas Mark 5 for 35-40 minutes, or until the apples are just beginning to go golden brown. As soon as the flan is removed from the oven, carefully brush the top with the warmed honey glaze.

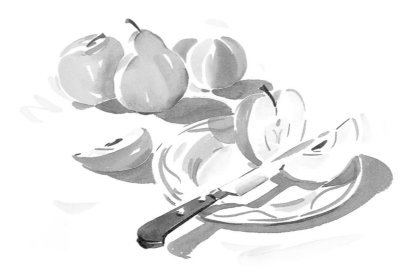

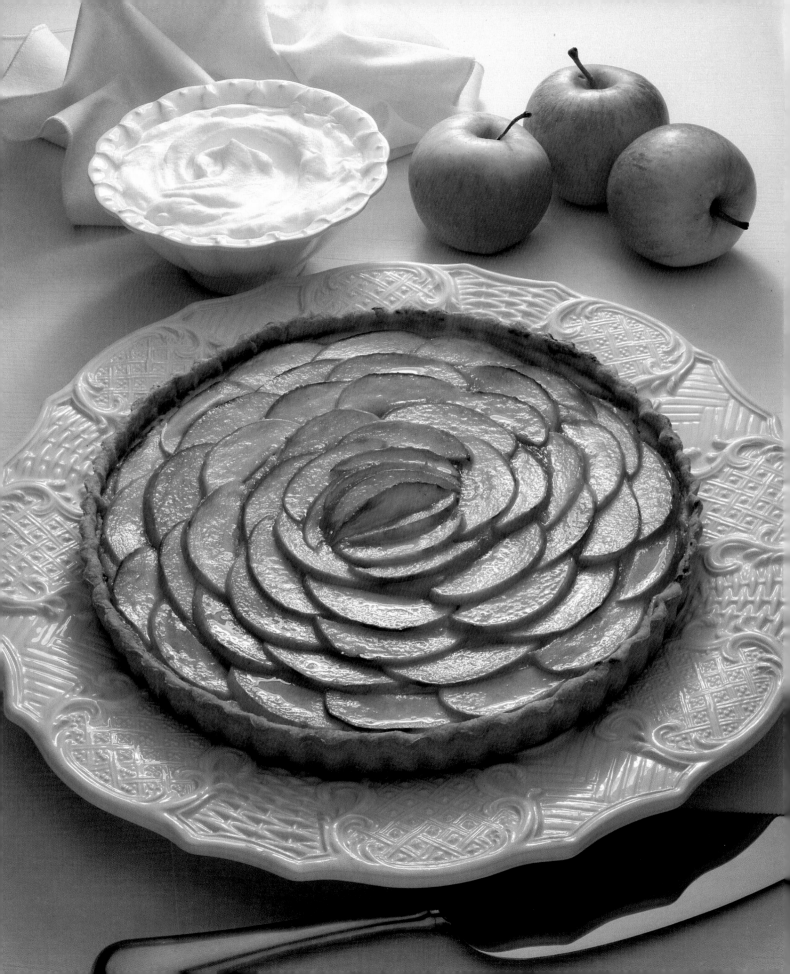

Exotic Fruit Salad

Preparation Time: 25 minutes, plus 1 hour chilling time **Serves:** 4-6

Mangoes are exceptionally sweet when ripe, and give this lovely fruit salad a natural tangy sweetness.

Ingredients
3 ripe peaches
3 kiwi fruits
1 large star fruit
120g/4oz fresh strawberries
2 well-ripened mangoes, each
   weighing about 340g/12oz

Juice of half a lime
150g/5oz redcurrants
Few strawberry leaves for decoration

Plunge the peaches into boiling water for a few seconds, then carefully peel away the skin using a sharp knife. Carefully cut them in half and remove the stone. Cut the halves into thin slices and arrange on a serving plate.

Peel the kiwi fruits and slice them crosswise to show their attractive colour. Trim away any dark pieces from the skin of the star fruit, cut the flesh into thin slices, and remove any small pips you may find. Leave the green stems on the strawberries and cut them in half lengthways. Arrange all the prepared fruit on the serving platter with the peaches.

Peel the mangoes and chop away the flesh from the large inner stone. Liquidize the chopped mango flesh with the lime juice and half of the redcurrants, then press the purée through a nylon sieve to remove the redcurrant skins and pips. Sprinkle the remaining redcurrants over the fruit on the serving platter, removing any hard stems or leaves as you do so. Pour the fruit purée evenly over the fruit salad, and chill for at least 1 hour before serving, decorated with the strawberry leaves.

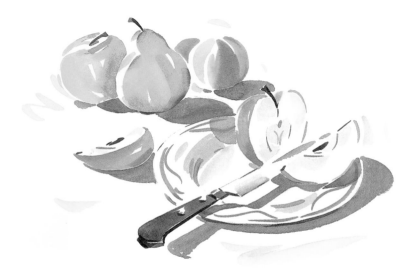

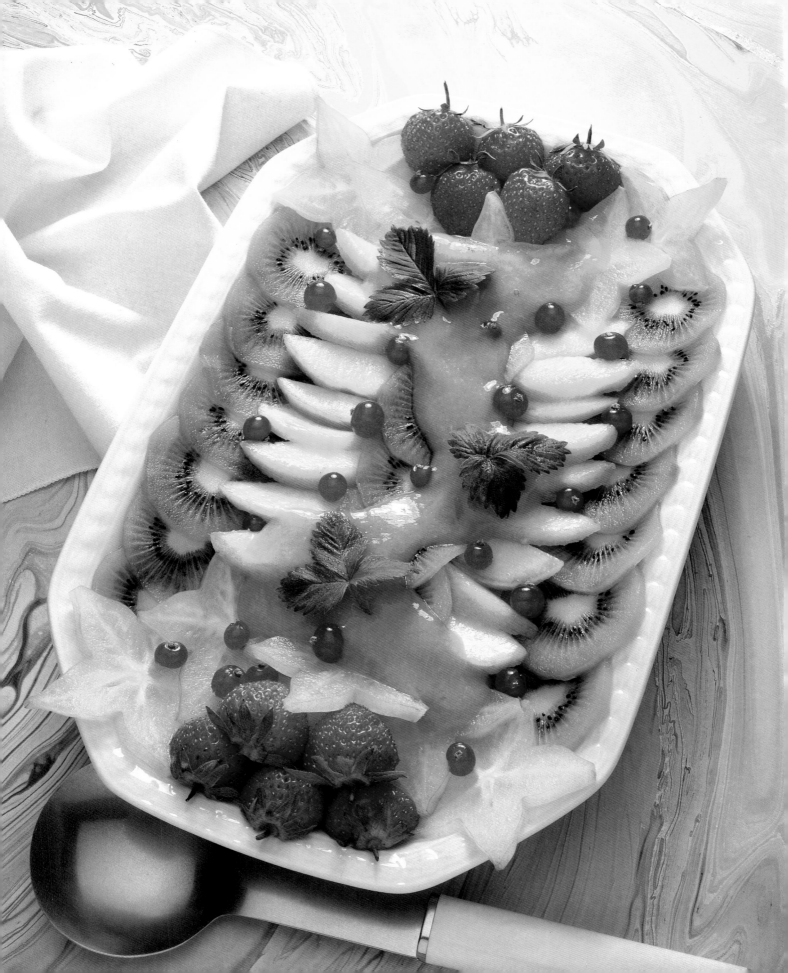

Prune, Apricot and Nut Flan

Preparation Time: 30 minutes, plus 4 hours soaking time
Cooking Time: 25 minutes **Serves:** 6-8

This sumptuous sweet tart has a nutty shortcake pastry for its base.

Ingredients

120g/4oz dried apricots
120g/4oz dried prunes
280ml/½ pint red wine, or dry cider
120g/4oz unsalted butter
60g/2oz soft brown sugar

120g/4oz plain flour
60g/2oz ground hazelnuts
3 tbsps finely chopped walnuts
2 tbsps clear honey, warmed

Put the apricots and prunes into a large bowl. Warm the wine or cider, and pour it over the dried fruit. Leave to stand for 4 hours minimum.

Put the butter and sugar into a large bowl and cream it together until it becomes light and fluffy. Gradually stir in the flour and ground hazelnuts. Knead the dough lightly until it is smooth, working in the chopped walnuts as you go. Press the shortcake dough evenly over the base of a 22.5cm/9-inch fluted loose-bottomed flan tin. Prick the surface of the dough with a fork and bake in a preheated oven, 190°C/375°F/Gas Mark 5, for 15 minutes.

Remove the prunes and apricots from the soaking liquid and drain them thoroughly on absorbent paper. Remove the shortcake from the oven and arrange the fruit over the hot shortcake. Cover the tart with aluminium foil and return to the oven for a further 10 minutes. Remove the shortcake carefully from its tin and arrange on a serving plate. While the shortcake is still hot, brush the fruit with the warmed honey to glaze.

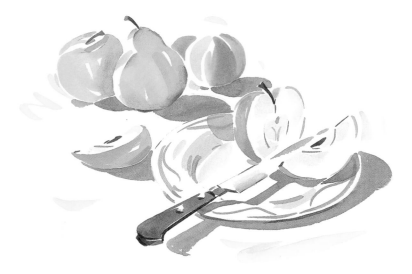

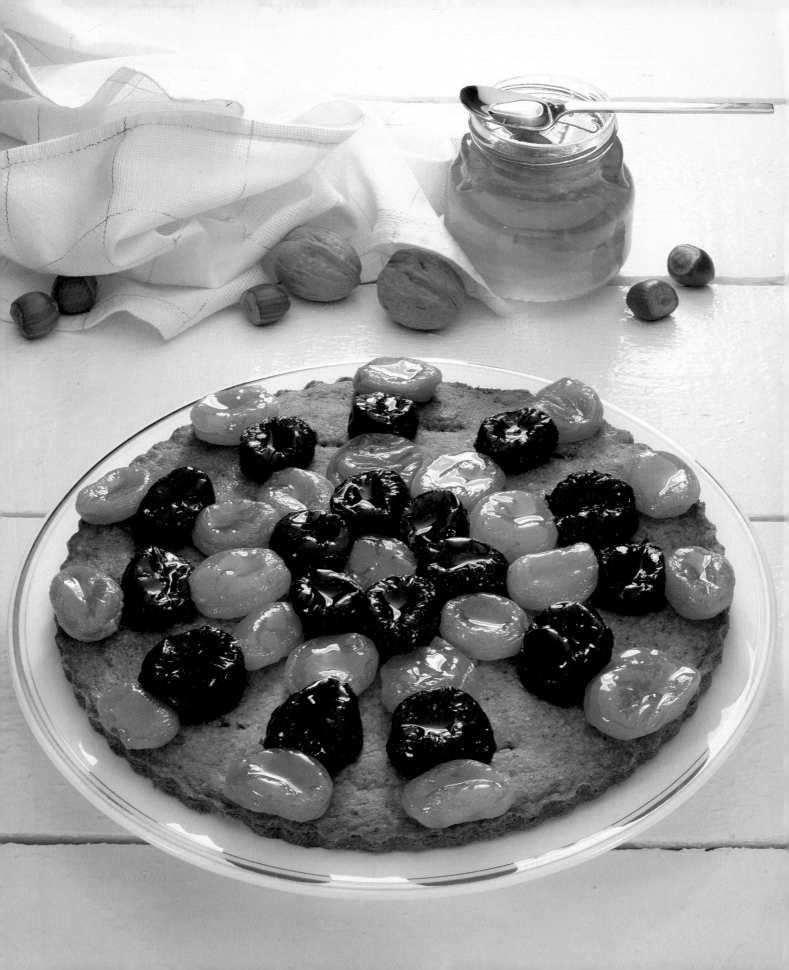

Carrot Cake

Preparation Time: 30 minutes **Cooking Time:** 45-50 minutes
Makes: 1 × 25cm/10-inch loaf

Carrots give a cake a delicious sweet flavour, as well as lots of vitamins and minerals. What better excuse do you need to indulge in this delicious tea-time treat?

Ingredients

180g/6oz butter
180g/6oz soft brown sugar
2 eggs, well beaten
225g/8oz plain wholemeal flour
1½ tsps bicarbonate of soda
½ tsp baking powder
¼ tsp ground cinnamon

¼ tsp ground nutmeg
½ tsp salt
225g/8oz peeled carrots, grated
90g/3oz raisins
60g/2oz finely chopped walnuts
¼ tsp cardamom seeds, crushed
Icing sugar for dredging

Cream the butter and sugar together until they are light and fluffy. Add the eggs a little at a time, beating well and adding a teaspoonful of the flour with each addition, to prevent the mixture from curdling. Put the remaining flour into a large bowl along with the bicarbonate of soda, baking powder, cinnamon, nutmeg and salt. Mix together well. Carefully fold the flour into the butter and egg mixture, mixing well to ensure that it is blended evenly. Add the carrots, raisins, nuts and cardamom seeds, beating the mixture well to blend evenly.

Lightly grease a 25cm/10-inch loaf tin and line the base with a piece of silicone paper. Pour the cake mixture into the loaf tin, and bake in a preheated oven 180°C/350°F/Gas Mark 4, for 45-50 minutes or until a fine metal skewer comes out clean when inserted into the centre of the cake. Cool the cake in its tin for 15 minutes before turning out onto a wire rack to cool completely. Dredge the cake with icing sugar just before serving.

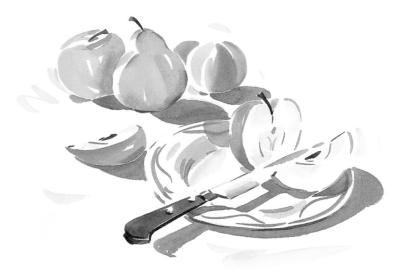

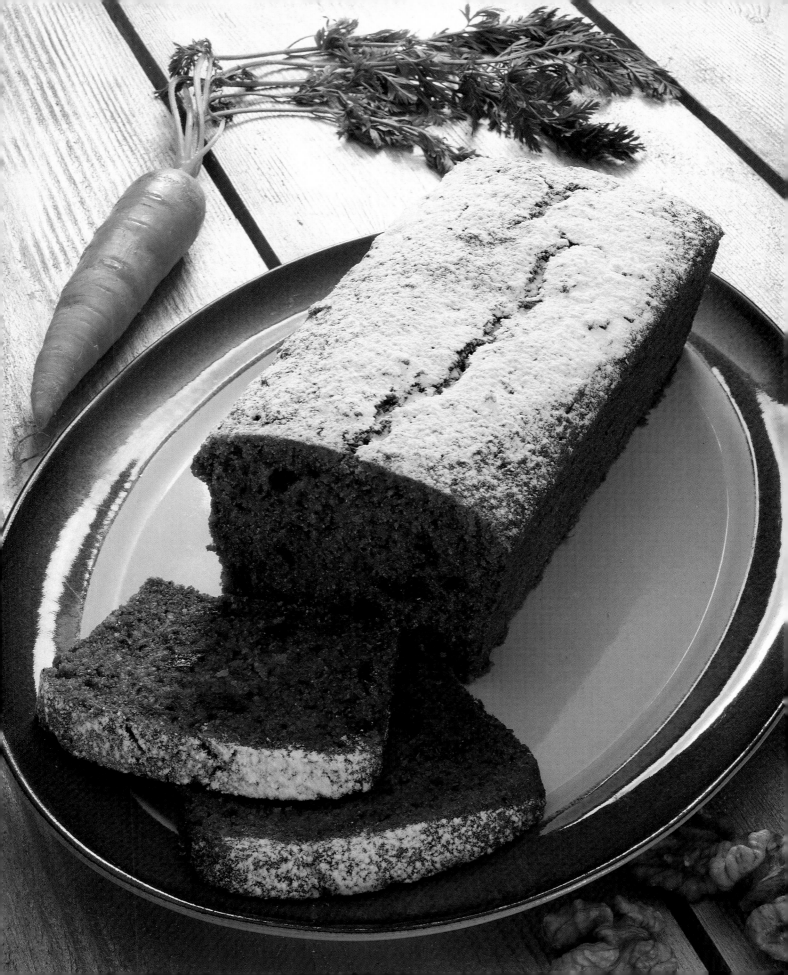

Strawberry Yogurt Ice

Preparation Time: 15 minutes, plus freezing time **Serves:** 4

Ice cream prepared with low fat natural yogurt and fresh fruit makes a delicious and healthy dessert.

Ingredients
225g/8oz fresh strawberries
280ml/½ pint low fat natural yogurt
2 tsps gelatin
2 tbsps boiling water

1 egg white
Liquid sweetener (optional)
Few fresh strawberries for decoration

Remove and discard the green stalks and leaves from the top of the strawberries. Roughly chop the fruit. Liquidize the strawberries with the yogurt until smooth. Sprinkle the gelatin over the boiling water in a small bowl. Stand the bowl into another, and pour in enough boiling water to come halfway up the sides of the dish. Allow the gelatin to stand, without stirring, until it has dissolved and the liquid has cleared. Pour the strawberry mixture into a bowl, and stir in the dissolved gelatin, mixing well to blend evenly. Place the bowl into a deep freeze and chill until just icy around the edges.

Remove the bowl from the deep freeze and beat until the chilled mixture is smooth. Return the bowl to the deep freeze and freeze once again in the same way. Remove the bowl from the deep freeze a second time, and whisk with an electric mixer until smooth. Whisk the egg white until it forms soft peaks and fold into the partially set strawberry mixture, carefully lifting and cutting the mixture to keep it light. Sweeten with a little liquid sweetener if necessary, then pour the strawberry ice into a shallow sided ice cream dish, and return to the freezer to freeze until completely set. Remove the ice cream 10 minutes before serving to soften slightly. Pile into serving dishes and decorate with a few extra strawberries.

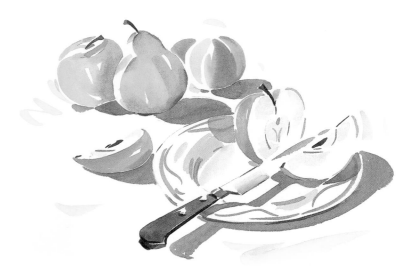

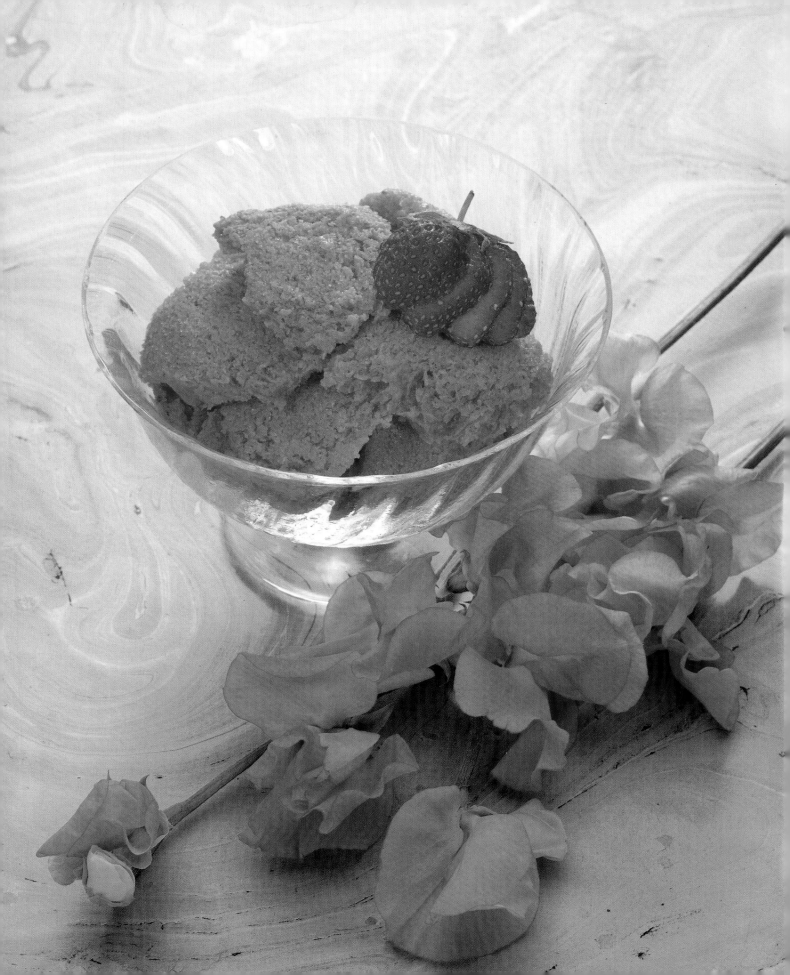

Andalusian Aubergines 56
Appetisers and Soups:
   Courgette Soup with Lemon 18
   Minestrone Soup 10
   Taramasalata 12
   Terrine of Spinach and
     Chicken 16
   Watercress Soup 14
Aubergine Bake 32
Beef with Pineapple and
   Peppers 40
Cakes and Desserts:
   Carrot Cake 66
   Exotic Fruit Salad 62
   Honey and Apple Tart 60
   Prune, Apricot and Nut Flan 64
   Strawberry Yogurt Ice 68
Carrot Cake 66
Casserole of Veal and
   Mushrooms 20
Cheese Salad 42
Chicken Liver Stir-Fry 52
Chicken with 'Burnt' Peppers and
   Coriander 58
Courgette Soup with Lemon 18
Dolmas 44
Exotic Fruit Salad 62
Fish and Seafood:
   Sole Kebabs 24
   Swedish Herrings 46
   Tarragon Grilled Red Mullet 38
Ham and Green Pepper
   Omelette 48
Honey and Apple Tart 60
Kidneys with Mustard
   Sauce 28
Lime Roasted Chicken 30
Liver with Onions 36
Minestrone Soup 10

Meat Dishes:
   Beef with Pineapple and
     Peppers 40
   Casserole of Veal and
     Mushrooms 20
   Ham and Green Pepper
     Omelette 48
   Kidneys with Mustard
     Sauce 28
   Liver with Onions 36
Poultry:
   Chicken Liver Stir-Fry 52
   Chicken with 'Burnt' Peppers and
     Coriander 58
   Lime Roasted Chicken 30
   Turkey Kebabs 50
Prune, Apricot and Nut Flan 64
Ratatouille 22
Salads:
   Cheese Salad 42
   Salade Paysanne 26
   Summer Pasta Salad 54
Salade Paysanne 26
Sole Kebabs 24
Strawberry Yogurt Ice 68
Summer Pasta Salad 54
Swedish Herrings 46
Taramasalata 12
Tarragon Grilled Red Mullet 38
Terrine of Spinach and Chicken 16
Turkey Kebabs 50
Vegetable Dishes:
   Andalusian Aubergines 56
   Aubergine Bake 32
   Dolmas 44
   Ratatouille 22
   Vegetable Kebabs 34
Vegetable Kebabs 34
Watercress Soup 14